Sex When You're Sick

Recent Titles in
Sex, Love, and Psychology
Judy Kuriansky, Series Editor

Relationship Sabotage: Unconscious Factors That Destroy Couples, Marriages, and Family
William J. Matta

The Praeger Handbook of Transsexuality: Changing Gender to Match Mindset
Rachel Ann Heath

America's War on Sex
Marty Klein

Teenagers, HIV, and AIDS: Insights from Youths Living with the Virus
Maureen E. Lyon and Lawrence J. D'Angelo, editors

Rock 'n' Roll Wisdom: What Psychologically Astute Lyrics Teach about Life and Love
Barry A. Farber

Sixty, Sexy, and Successful: A Guide for Aging Male Baby Boomers
Robert Schwalbe, PhD

Managing Menopause Beautifully: Physically, Emotionally, and Sexually
Dona Caine-Francis

New Frontiers in Men's Sexual Health: Understanding Erectile Dysfunction and the
Revolutionary New Treatments
Kamal A. Hanash, MD

Sexuality Education: Past, Present, and Future (4 volumes)
Elizabeth Schroeder, EdD, MSW, and Judy Kuriansky, PhD, editors

SEX WHEN YOU'RE SICK

Reclaiming Sexual Health after Illness or Injury

Anne Katz

Sex, Love, and Psychology
Judy Kuriansky, Series Editor

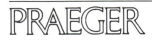

Westport, Connecticut
London

Library of Congress Cataloging-in-Publication Data

Katz, Anne.
Sex when you're sick : reclaiming sexual health after illness or injury / Anne Katz.
    p. cm. — (Sex, love, and psychology, ISSN 1554–222X)
    Includes index.
    ISBN 978–0–313–37233–9 (alk. paper)
    1. Sexual disorders. 2. Sex. 3. Sex (Psychology) I. Title.
RC556.K35 2009
616.6'9—dc22   2008053794

British Library Cataloguing in Publication Data is available.

Library of Congress Catalog Card Number: 2008053794

ISBN: 978–0–313–37233–9
ISSN: 1554–222X

First published in 2009

Praeger Publishers, 88 Post Road West, Westport, CT 06881
An imprint of Greenwood Publishing Group, Inc.
www.praeger.com

Printed in the United States of America

The paper used in this book complies with the
Permanent Paper Standard issued by the National
Information Standards Organization (Z39.48-1984).

10 9 8 7 6 5 4 3 2 1

To Alan
husband, friend, supporter, playmate, travel companion,
physician, researcher, critic
Love

CONTENTS

Series Foreword   ix
Dr. Judy Kuriansky

Acknowledgments   xi

PART I   THE BASICS

1. Introduction   3

2. How Things Work   8

PART II   SEXUALITY AND ILLNESS

3. Sexuality across the Life Span   25

4. Sexuality in Medical Disease   34

5. Sexuality in Surgical Disease   60

6. Sexuality in Mental Illness   71

7. Sexuality following Combat Injury   82

8. Sexuality following Spinal Cord Injury   91

9. Sexuality in Men with Cancer   97

10. Sexuality in Women with Cancer   115

11. Sexuality and Cancer in Both Men and Women   133

12. Sexual Dysfunction   145

Index   161

SERIES FOREWORD

Sex is good for your health—which is why this book is essential for anyone whose own health or that of a loved one is threatened. The message is crucial—that injury or illness requires adjustments in life, for sure, but does not equal the end of loving. All too often, an injury or an illness is so troubling or traumatic that people put aside that important part of their life—intimacy—when that is the very part of their life that could, and should, be continued.

I remember the early days of sexology, when I was first learning about the impact on sexual functioning of various medical conditions. Researchers and health experts contributed to a pioneer academic book about the topic. At that time, in distilling the complicated information for the public on my television reports and radio call-in advice shows, I set forth my "3 F's" of healthy sexuality in the face of illness: Get the Facts, express Feelings, and continue aFfection.

How wonderful now to read this comprehensive book, which is so accessible not only to the profession but to the vast public, and see those 3 F's so clearly and positively laid out. As Dr. Katz draws on her wealth of experience in the field of health, she spells out the facts about various common injuries and illnesses in clear detail, explains the feelings that patients and loved ones may have and the sexual problems that may arise, and then gives helpful "solutions" presenting advice on how to go about resuming and restoring healthy sexuality.

Since millions of men and women in America—and around the world—confront a diagnosis affecting their physical health, they will be reassured in reading this book that their sexual health does not have to suffer. In this way, this book offers hope to so many, as they courageously face their future.

Dr. Judy Kuriansky

ACKNOWLEDGMENTS

Writing books is mostly keeping one's bum in the chair when friends and colleagues are socializing and taking vacations. For me, writing has always meant very early mornings alone in my office while most of the rest of my world sleeps. But writing is also supported by people who facilitate the work, and I have three people to thank for this. The first is Ruth Holmberg, the librarian at CancerCare Manitoba. Ruth has photocopied and printed thousands of articles, sometimes at very short notice and always with a smile. Second, my husband Alan, who has read every word of this book and learned more than he probably needs to know. And finally my thanks to Geoff Hayes, artist and friend, who never blinked when I presented him with photos and illustrations of body parts he has only seen in private and asked him to draw them for this book, only better!

Part I

THE BASICS

Chapter One

INTRODUCTION

This book was written to explore something that has the potential to affect each and every one of us when we become ill. Experts around the world agree that sexuality is an important part of the quality of life. They know this because men and women tell them that this is so. For most of us, sexuality may not be the most important factor in our lives, but when it is threatened, we notice that something important has gone out of our lives. Challenges to our health are inevitable, and with ill health comes a change in the quality of life. If we are lucky, this change will be temporary and minor. If we are not that fortunate, we will have to learn to live an altered life.

This book has two sections. In the first you will read about the basics of human sexuality: how things work and how we grow as sexual beings across the life span. The second section describes various illnesses and how they alter or threaten our sexuality. The chapters in this section contain the stories of men and women who have the condition under discussion. These chapters tell their stories and discuss what happened when they tried to seek help or just ignored what was going on. You will meet their partners and family members, all of whom are affected by the illness, surgery, or injury. In each chapter, solutions are presented to the sexual problems highlighted by the stories. There are some happy endings, but for many, sexual problems persist and may eventually cause harm to personal relationships.

SO WHY READ THIS BOOK?

This book will inform you (and your partner) about the sexual challenges that may result from a particular illness or injury you are experiencing. But you probably know about this already, because you are living it! This book will explain *why* this is happening and also what you can do to get help. But there are three important steps along the way.

The first step is that you need to acknowledge that this is happening to you. That can be difficult at times. Sometimes we cope with loss by ignoring what has been lost or telling ourselves it doesn't matter. But it does matter! Sexuality is important because it plays various roles in our inner life as well as in our social life. Our sexuality plays a role in how we see ourselves as men and women. The body parts involved in sexual activity are the outward proof of ourselves as men and women. Our sexuality is also an important part of our relationships. Sexuality plays a role in making and keeping our primary relationship with a partner or spouse an intimate one where we share the deepest part of ourselves.

The second step is to talk to your partner or spouse about what you are feeling and thinking. This may not be easy; it is very difficult for many of us to find the words to explain that we are not feeling things the same way or that we can't do something in the bedroom anymore or we don't want to. So often we avoid this conversation or the opportunity of having sex; we go to bed before or after our partner or spouse, or we pick a fight to avoid having sex. There are many strategies that can be used to deny or prevent an honest discussion. Why do we do this? Because many of us have never been challenged in this way before and we don't know what to say; we just don't have the words. Many of us have never talked out loud about "those" parts of our bodies or what we do with them. We are embarrassed or ashamed or don't want to hurt our partner's feelings. So we don't talk about it, we don't share our fears, we remain silent.

The third step is to get help. This can be daunting, because where do you go for this help? How do you find out who to talk to? In a perfect world, the health care provider that you are seeing for your illness will have told you what to expect in terms of sexual changes. She will have asked you on numerous occasions if you are having any problems in that part of your life. But this is not a perfect world, and your physician or nurse may never have asked you or told you. Why is this so, if sexuality is so important? Your health care provider is a person just like you. He may not have had any or much education about human sexuality. He may be as embarrassed as you to say the words. He may be shy or may not want to seem nosy or appear to be prying into a private part of your life. But your health care provider has a responsibility to provide care to the whole of you. And sexuality is part of you and your life. Your provider needs to tell you about the sexual consequences of your illness or its treatment in the same way as she tells you about the side effects of drugs or the complications of surgery.

But you may have to ask your provider first. We know that health care providers are willing to talk about sexuality if the patient asks first. And patients want to talk about it, if the health care provider is open to listening! The result is a deafening silence; the patient doesn't ask and the provider doesn't indicate that he is open to talking about it. This book is intended to do two things: to provide you with information on what may happen to you if you become ill and to explain to you why this is happening. You may find that this amount of information is enough. The book will also give you the words to go to your health care provider and say: "I read this book and it said that someone like me with my condition may have the following sexual problems. And it suggested what can be done about it. I would like to talk to you about this."

WHAT THIS BOOK IS ALL ABOUT

This book presents a head-to-toe overview of how sexuality is affected by illness. It is divided into two parts. The first part lays the groundwork for understanding human sexuality. Chapter 2 describes the basics of sexual functioning by describing both male and female anatomy as well as the hormonal basis of sexual functioning. In this chapter you will also learn about the way we conceive of how the sexual response cycle works. Chapter 3 describes sexual development across the life span. There are key milestones that must be achieved if a person is to become a healthy sexual being, and these milestones occur in the four distinct developmental stages of adolescence, the childbearing years, midlife, and old age.

The next section of the book contains eight chapters. Each chapter details conditions that affect sexual functioning. In chapter 4, you will learn about sexuality and medical conditions. Certain medical conditions have a direct effect on sexual functioning. These conditions are extremely common and occur across the life span but are particularly prevalent in middle-aged and older adults. These conditions include heart disease, multiple sclerosis, arthritis, Sjogren's disease, lung disease, and diabetes. Sexuality is also affected by HIV/AIDS, renal disease, incontinence, and obesity.

Chapter 5 deals with common surgeries that men and women undergo and the sexual consequences of these surgeries. Hysterectomy is the second most common surgery performed on women, and it has very real sexual side effects. The chapter also describes the sexual consequences of surgery to the colon. Cardiac surgery and orthopedic surgery also have the potential to cause significant sexual problems. Finally, this chapter describes the sexual side effects of surgery performed to treat benign prostatic hypertrophy, a condition in which the prostate enlarges and causes urinary problems.

Chapter 6 describes mental illness and its effect on sexuality. The chapter opens with a discussion of depression and anxiety, both of which can affect sexuality. People with obsessive compulsive disorder also experience sexual consequences, often due to the medications prescribed to treat this condition. Schizophrenia is a more serious mental illness that has profound effects on sexual functioning. People who abuse recreational drugs and alcohol also have sexual problems as a result of their drug and alcohol abuse. Finally, the chapter describes some of the sexual issues for those with intellectual disabilities.

Chapter 7 describes the sexual consequences of combat injury. Many of our service members return from war zones with significant injuries to their bodies and minds. Amputation and burns cause significant trauma to tissues as well as to body image; this affects sexuality directly. Traumatic brain injury also affects sexual functioning and may have a profound effect on the sexual partner. Posttraumatic stress disorder has wide-ranging effects on mood and behavior, and sexual functioning for both the service member and the partner can be profoundly altered by the personality changes and depression that are part of this syndrome.

Chapter 8 describes what happens when someone receives a spinal cord injury. Hundreds of thousands of people are injured in accidents each year. Spinal cord injury devastates the lives of those affected, including their sexual lives. Both men and women are affected, and the degree of sexual damage is related to the place in the spinal cord where the trauma is located as well as to the degree of damage to the spinal cord tissue.

Chapters 9, 10, and 11 describe the sexual consequences of cancer and its treatments. All of those who experience a cancer diagnosis and then go through treatment will experience either short-term or permanent alterations to their sexual lives. Cancers that are unique to men present challenges, as these cancers directly affect male sexual functioning. In chapter 9, cancers that affect men are discussed; cancer of the prostate, penis, and testicle will be described along with their sexual side effects and solutions to these problems. Chapter 10 details the common cancers that women experience and their sexual side effects. These common women's cancers include breast cancer and the gynecological cancers including cancer of the cervix, vulva, and vagina. Chapter 11 deals with cancers that affect both men and women. While it may seem obvious that someone with breast, gynecological, or prostate cancer will suffer sexual consequences from the treatment, other forms of cancer, including the childhood cancers, also present challenges. Chapter 11 describes the sexual consequences of bladder cancer and cancer of the colon and rectum. The adolescent with cancer is also discussed.

Chapter 12 presents an overview of both male and female sexual dysfunction with suggestions for treatment and coping strategies. Although there is a formal definition and classification of this dysfunction in the medical literature, others suggest that sexual dysfunction can be seen in the context of lack of knowledge and poor access to resources. An alternative model of sexual dysfunction is presented to illustrate this.

SO WHAT NOW?

Start at the beginning of this book; read chapters 2 and 3 to set in place the groundwork for what comes next. Then you may want to search for the particular illness that you have or your partner has. Read the story of the person in that chapter; he may not experience exactly what you are going through, but you will learn from his story. And then continue reading. . . .

Chapter Two

HOW THINGS WORK

Human sexuality is complex. What is it? A simple definition of human sexuality is the quality or state of being sexual. It is also defined as sexual activity and the expression of sexual receptivity or interest. It is more fully described as the ways in which human beings experience and express themselves as sexual beings. Awareness of ourselves as females and males is part of our sexuality. The capacity we have for erotic experiences and responses is also a part of our sexuality. Our sexuality is an essential part of who we are, whether or not we ever engage in sexual intercourse or sexual fantasy, or even if we lose sensation in our genitals because of injury. Sexuality is also seen as a central aspect of being human throughout life, encompassing sex, gender, identities and roles, sexual orientation, eroticism, pleasure, intimacy, and reproduction. Our view of ourselves and others as sexual beings is influenced by cultural, ethnic, and religious beliefs and practices.

Sexuality also encompasses our relationships with others and the way we are perceived by others as sexual beings. Sexuality is sometimes spoken of as *intimacy,* and this word is often used as a euphemism for sexual activity. In the truest sense of the word, intimacy involves a close and open relationship with a partner in which mutual disclosure of thoughts and feelings occurs.

The World Health Organization describes sexuality as "a central aspect of being human throughout life," encompassing "sex, gender identities and roles, sexual orientation, eroticism, pleasure, intimacy, and reproduction. Sexuality is experienced and expressed in thoughts, fantasies, desires, beliefs, attitudes, values, behaviors, practices, roles, and relationships. While sexuality can include all of these dimensions, not all of them are always experienced or expressed. Sexuality is influenced by the interaction of biological, psychological, social, economic, political, cultural, ethical, legal, historical, religious, and spiritual factors" (WHO 2004). These definitions contrast with what we understand by the term *sexual functioning;* this is what we *do* as sexual beings. Sexual functioning is sexual behavior, and this sets the norm for what is supposed to happen. Any change from the norm is regarded as sexual dysfunction.

A basic component of sexuality is the structure and function of sexual and reproductive organs that act together with and under the influence of hormones. The brain plays an important role as well, through cognition, emotion, motivation, and memory. We have learned a lot about human sexuality over the past 50 years, and our understanding has increased, but there are still aspects of sexuality that we do not talk about, and these include the effects of disease. Let us start by talking about how things work, in order to lay the groundwork for an understanding of how illness may affect our sexual lives.

SEXUAL ANATOMY

For women, the sexual organs are the breasts, the pubic mound, the vulva (made up of the clitoris, the labia majora and minora [outer and inner lips], and the entrance to the vagina), the vagina, and the cervix, and internally the uterus and uterine tubes. The ovaries produce the hormones that influence sexual functioning.

The breasts are regarded as secondary sex characteristics, and they grow and develop during the years of puberty. The breasts are made up of special tissue called mammary glands, which produce milk, and of fat, which gives the breasts their size and shape. Each breast has a nipple that is surrounded by a colored area called the areola. The nipples and areolae are well supplied with nerve endings that are important for sexual arousal.

The pubic mound is a pad of fatty tissue over the pubic bone and is covered by hair from puberty. This pad of fat protects the woman and her partner from feeling pain during intercourse, where the pubic bones of both partners would bang into each other. The outer lips of the vulva (called the labia majora) are two thick folds of skin that run backward to the entrance to the vagina from the pubic mound in the front. They cover and protect the inner lips (the labia minora), the opening of the urethra (which carries urine from the bladder), and the entrance to the vagina. This area is richly supplied with nerve endings and blood and swells during sexual excitement.

The clitoris, which is found where the labia meet in the front, is a complex system of nerve endings. The body of the clitoris is about half an inch wide and one to two inches long. Two large wings (called *crura* in Latin), which are two to four inches long, extend sideways from the body under the outer lips. Two other structures made of the same erectile tissue form the internal structure of the clitoris and are called the bulbs of the clitoris. All these tissues are richly supplied with nerves and blood vessels and play an important role in sexual arousal. The only part of the clitoris that is visible is partially covered by a hood (see Figures 2.1 and 2.2).

The vaginal opening lies between the opening of the urethra in the front and the anus behind. The vagina itself is a tube that extends upward and backward and is about three to five inches in length. At rest, the walls touch one another along their length. The vaginal walls are lined with a mucosal layer that is richly supplied with blood vessels but has few nerve endings other than in the lower one-third close to the entrance. The mucosal layer has numerous folds and secretes an acidic fluid that keeps the vaginal membranes moist.

The cervix is the internal entrance to the uterus (or womb) and is found at the top of the vagina. The cervix itself secretes fluid and on either side is found a bundle of nerves and blood vessels that supply the pelvic tissues. The uterus is a pear-shaped muscular organ; the uterine tubes extend from each side of the uterus with their ends lying close to the ovaries. The ovaries produce the sexual hormones including estrogen, progesterone, and testosterone.

The external male sexual organs are the penis and the scrotum. The internal organs are the testicles, the vas deferens, the seminal vesicles, the Cowper's

Figure 2.1
Female sexual organs: frontal view. Illustration by Geoff Hayes.

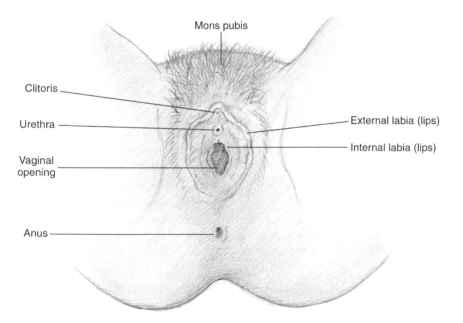

Figure 2.2
Female sexual organs: side view. Illustration by Geoff Hayes.

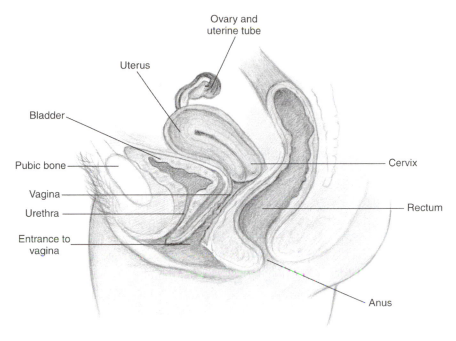

glands, and the prostate. The penis consists of three cylinders of spongy tissue that run along its length. Two of these are called the corpora cavernosa and they lie on either side of the urethra (the tube through which urine passes); these fill with blood when the man is aroused. The other cylinder of spongy tissue is called the corpus spongiosum. It contains the urethra and widens at the end of the penis to become the glans or head of the penis. The head of the penis is covered loosely by the foreskin; this is sometimes surgically removed in infancy (circumcision). The base of the penis extends deeper into the pelvis, where it ends and is anchored to the pelvic bones.

The scrotum is a sac of tissue that contains the two testicles; it is covered in pubic hair after puberty. The testicles lie in their own compartments in the scrotum and are held in place by the spermatic cords containing the vas deferens—through which sperm travel—nerves, and blood vessels. The cremaster muscles raise and lower the testicles in response to sexual stimulation and temperature changes.

The internal organs include the testes, which are the site of sperm and testosterone production. Other internal organs include the seminal vesicles, which are connected to the prostate gland and produce a fluid rich in fructose that nourishes the sperm. The prostate gland manufactures prostatic fluid, which together with the sperm and fluid from the seminal vesicles forms the ejaculate. The Cowper's glands (bulbourethral glands) lie below the prostate gland. During arousal, the fluid from these glands often appears at the tip of the penis prior to ejaculation and is known as pre-ejaculatory fluid (or pre-cum) (see Figures 2.3. and 2.4).

HORMONAL INFLUENCES

The secretion of sex hormones is regulated by the brain; the sex hormones are produced by the ovaries in women and the testes in men, in response to the other hormones circulating in the bloodstream. The ovaries produce estrogen, progesterone, and small amounts of testosterone. The testes produce testosterone. These hormones are important in the development of secondary sex characteristics, as well as in various aspects of sexual functioning. Another hormone, prolactin, is secreted by the pituitary gland at the base of the brain and also plays a role in sexual functioning.

Figure 2.3
Male sexual organs: frontal view. Illustration by Geoff Hayes.

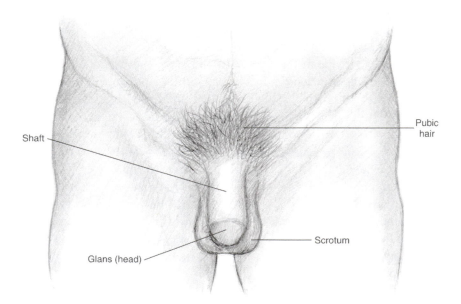

Figure 2.4
Male sexual organs: side view. Illustration by Geoff Hayes

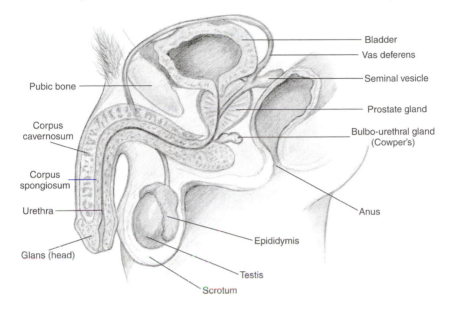

Estrogen is often called the hormone of arousal and plays an important role in the lubrication of the vagina. After menopause, much of the ovarian production of estrogen stops, but a small amount is still made in fatty tissue. Progesterone is also made in the ovaries and plays an important role in the regulation of the menstrual cycle, along with estrogen. Women also produce small amounts of testosterone in the ovaries and also in the adrenal glands that lie on top of the kidneys. Testosterone is known as the hormone of desire, and it certainly seems to be an important factor in male sexual functioning, but the role it plays for women is less clear. Testosterone and estrogen are thought to play a role in the way sexual sensations are perceived in the brains of women. Testosterone production in the ovaries declines sharply in women in their 20s and 30s and does not change much after menopause, with the ovaries still producing the hormone.

In men, testosterone is produced mainly in the testicles with a small amount coming from the adrenal glands. Prolactin plays a role in controlling the production of testosterone; high levels of prolactin reduce the amount of testosterone and decrease desire in men. Men have a small amount of estrogen in their bodies; this is produced in the testicles and also when testosterone is broken down in the body.

THE BRAIN

We often talk about the brain as being the largest sex organ in the body. There's a good reason for this. The brain is involved in almost all sexual thoughts and activity. The brain recognizes sexual thoughts and fantasies and sends messages to the sexual organs; they respond by filling with blood. This is what arousal is all about. The brain also responds to sexual touch and controls the interpretation of sexual touching as stimulating or not, and as pleasurable or not.

THE SEXUAL RESPONSE CYCLE

For many years we had little or no understanding of the human sexual response cycle. It was just not talked about at all. But a team of sex researchers changed all that in the 1960s. Drs. William Masters and Virginia Johnson performed a series of studies suggesting that there were four distinct stages in the human sexual response (see Figures 2.5 and 2.6). These were described as taking place one after the other and were essentially the same for both men and women. The four stages Masters and Johnson described were excitement, plateau, orgasm, and resolution.

In the excitement phase, heart rate and blood pressure increase. In women, this is accompanied by swelling of the breasts and a reddish flush over the chest and neck. The nipples also become erect. Blood flows into the tissues of the genital area and the clitoris enlarges. The outer lips also swell and flatten out while the inner lips grow larger. The upper two-thirds of the vagina balloon out and grow much bigger than in the resting state. The walls of the vagina also thicken and secrete fluid that lubricates the vagina.

In men during the excitement phase, we see a hardening of the penis as blood flows into the two cylinders of spongy tissue. The skin of the scrotum also grows thicker. The testicles enlarge and move inward toward the body.

The plateau phase is a state of advanced arousal. Heart rate and blood pressure continue to increase, and breathing becomes more rapid. Some people experience involuntary facial movements and the hands and feet also move by themselves. During this phase, the entrance and lower third of the vagina swell while the upper two-thirds continue to balloon outward. The uterus moves into an upright position. The inner lips become engorged with blood and may even change color. The clitoris shortens and may almost disappear under the clitoral hood. The breasts continue to swell and the areolae also grow, making the nipples appear flatter. In men, the testicles continue to enlarge and move into the body. The head of the penis changes to a darker color, and a small amount of fluid from the Cowper's glands may appear at the tip of the penis.

The orgasmic phase is one of intense muscle contractions and pleasurable sensations felt over the whole body. Many of the major muscles in the body also

Figure 2.5
Male sexual response cycle. Illustration by Geoff Hayes.

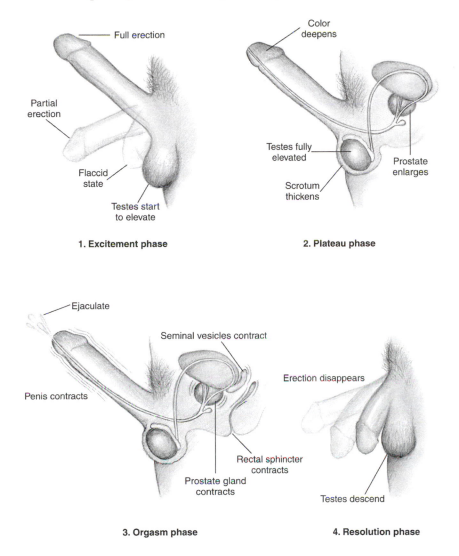

contract. In women, the uterus and the anal sphincter contract. The muscles of the pelvic floor also contract between three and fifteen times during orgasm. The male orgasm includes two stages. The first stage involves the movement of seminal fluid into the penis via the vas deferens, the prostate gland, and the seminal vesicles and ejaculatory ducts. These contract and close off the entry to the bladder, which lies just above the prostate gland; this prevents semen

Figure 2.6
Female sexual response cycle. Illustration by Geoff Hayes.

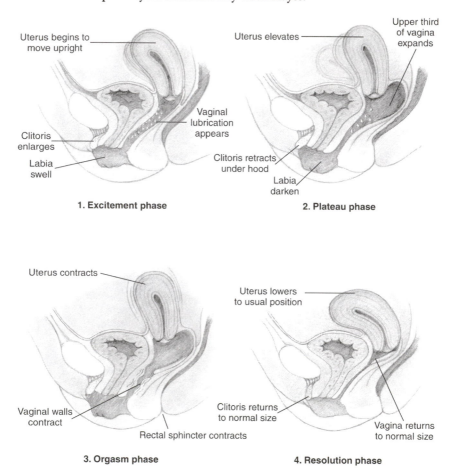

Uterus begins to move upright

Vaginal lubrication appears

Clitoris enlarges

Labia swell

1. Excitement phase

Uterus elevates

Upper third of vagina expands

Clitoris retracts under hood

Labia darken

2. Plateau phase

Uterus contracts

Vaginal walls contract

Rectal sphincter contracts

3. Orgasm phase

Uterus lowers to usual position

Clitoris returns to normal size

Vagina returns to normal size

4. Resolution phase

from mixing with urine. When this fluid enters the penis, it is experienced by the man as the point at which he can no longer control either the sensation of orgasm or the passage of semen to the outside. The second stage of male orgasm occurs when the semen is pushed along the urethra to the outside; this is called ejaculation.

The resolution phase encompasses the return of the body to its prearousal state. Blood leaves the sexual organs, muscle tension dissipates, and blood pressure and heart rate return to normal. In men, this phase is followed by a refractory period in which orgasm and ejaculation are not possible. In young men, this phase may last only a few minutes. As men age, the refractory period lasts longer, and older men may not be able to have another orgasm for many hours or even days. Women do not have a refractory period and are sometimes able to have multiple orgasms in the same encounter.

This description of how things work formed the basis of our understanding of human sexuality, but an important part of the body was missing. The brain was not included in this model. This was remedied by the work of one of Masters and Johnson's students, Helen Singer Kaplan. She suggested that a three-stage model comprising desire, excitement, and orgasm more adequately depicted the human sexual response cycle. Singer Kaplan's model included the brain's role in emotion and cognition, which together lead to a subjective feeling of desire. In her model, excitement is described as it was described by Masters and Johnson: blood flow causes lubrication in women and erections in men. Orgasm according to Singer Kaplan's model is a series of intense muscle contractions and pleasurable feelings. Singer Kaplan's model was not intended to be linear, and she thought that the three stages could be experienced independently of each other. But many people interpret her model as being linear, perhaps because it is presented that way, with desire leading to excitement and ending with orgasm.

Zilbergeld and Ellison suggest a five-and-a-half-part model with both physiological and psychological components. These components are independent of each other and comprise the following stages: interest, arousal, physiological readiness, orgasm, and satisfaction. Interest corresponds to desire as described by Singer Kaplan. Arousal is much the same as described by Masters and Johnson, with increased blood supply to the sexual organs. Zilbergeld and Ellison, however, describe a stage of physiological readiness (lubrication for the woman and erection for the man), without which intercourse is not possible. Orgasm then follows and has two parts: the physiological, in which muscles contract, and a second, subjective part in which pleasurable sensations are felt. The final stage of their model is that of satisfaction, which is both cognitive and emotional.

A more recent description of the female sexual response cycle is presented by Rosemary Basson. This model has a heavy emphasis on psycho-emotional processes. It is circular and does not suggest that one phase comes before or after another. Basson suggests that women have many different reasons to be receptive to the sexual advances of their partner. Feelings of emotional intimacy and well-being are important, as is the lack of the negative feelings that often follow avoidance of sexual activity. If the woman is receptive and advances are made in an appropriate context, it is then that the woman's brain processes what she is thinking and feeling, and this may be recognized as feelings of arousal and perhaps even desire for sexual activity. If sexual satisfaction occurs, and this does not mean that the woman necessarily has an orgasm, then the woman is more likely to be both receptive and motivated the next time. Basson suggests that many women are satisfied if they see that their partner is satisfied, and they are happy to feel emotionally close to their partner; they do not need to have an orgasm. In this model, desire or libido can be experienced at different stages of the cycle and is not necessarily the first stage as depicted by Singer Kaplan.

HUMANS AS SEXUAL BEINGS

Human beings like to do things the same way over and over again. We are creatures of habit for the most part, although novelty is exciting for many. This applies to our sex lives too. We find something that works and we do it over and over, in the same way. The ways in which we act and react in our sexual lives are referred to as our sexual scripts. These scripts are learned behaviors and meanings that we employ in our sexual lives. We may have an individual sexual script and also one that we use when we are with our partner(s). These scripts dictate what we do, with whom, when, and how. We learn these scripts from a variety of sources. We learn from our parents and the extent of the affection they showed and show toward each other. Our peer group plays a role, especially in adolescence. The media are highly influential and can sometimes supersede the messages we get from our parents about being sexual, if we have received any messages from them! Our religious groups also help to influence our sexual scripts. There are as many sexual scripts as there are people and their relationships. Our present partner and his or her own sexual scripts may change what we do when we are with our present partner as opposed to a previous partner.

Here is a sexual script that depicts a fairly narrow range of sexual activity: John and June are a couple in their mid-forties. They were sexually inexperienced when they met 25 years ago. Sex usually takes place on a Saturday night, after they have watched the late news. They both wear pajamas when they get into bed, and after June switches off the bedside light, John spends a few moments touching her breasts while they kiss. After a few moments, June reaches into John's pajama bottoms and strokes his penis. He is usually partially erect when she starts, and within a few moments he is fully erect. He asks her if she is "ready" and she usually replies that she is. He gets on top of her and after three or four minutes of thrusting, he ejaculates. He lies on top of her for a few minutes, and then she tries to move a bit and he returns to his side of the bed and falls asleep. She gets up and goes to the bathroom to clean up, and when she returns to their room, he is snoring faintly. While she may not be fulfilled by this activity, she would not suggest anything else. That would be outside their sexual script.

Other sexual scripts may be more inventive and creative. Brad and Sue have been together for more than 10 years. They have never married, believing that marriage stifles the sexual tension in a relationship. To maintain a high level of sexual tension, their sexual scripts usually include some form of surprise and novelty. For example, Brad works from home and every now and then he prepares something special for Sue. Once he waited behind the door at the time that Sue would usually come home. When she entered the house, Brad stepped out from behind the door and bound and gagged her, then took her into the dining room where she remained tied to the table for the next couple of hours. Brad teased and stimulated her with a variety of household items: a tea towel from the kitchen and hot wax from the candelabra that usually sat on the dining room table.

Some people use the same script over and over again; if this results in satisfaction for both partners then it may not be a bad thing. There is comfort in familiarity and consistency. But when illness challenges these well-established scripts, many couples are not able to adapt and modify or change their sexual script so as to still be able to enjoy each other and achieve satisfaction. This can lead to a great deal of frustration and distress.

TALKING ABOUT SEX

For many of us, sex is really difficult to talk about. We can joke about it, but to have a really meaningful conversation about this intimate topic, even with the person we are sexually active with, is really challenging. It is also difficult to talk to our health care provider about it. Providers usually don't ask, and we don't raise the topic.

We should be able to talk to them about an important part of life. But we don't raise the topic and neither do they. Why is that? It may be that we are shy or don't have the words to ask, or think that we don't know the right words. We may be afraid of embarrassing ourselves by using a slang term or we may think we are the only person in the world who has ever had this problem or feeling. Or we may think that the doctor or nurse doesn't have time or will think we are weird. Well, guess what? Our health care providers are people too, and they may not ask about this part of our lives because they are embarrassed or don't want to seem to be intruding into a private area. They may be wary of talking to a patient who is much older than themselves, or they may think (erroneously) that older people don't have sex or don't want to talk about it. Believe it or not, health care providers may have had very little education on human sexuality in their medical or nursing programs. These are not excuses; they are just the plain facts. Most health care providers will tell you that if the patient asks them about something to do with sexuality, they would be happy to talk about it. So the patient doesn't ask and the health care provider doesn't ask and the result is a deafening silence.

If you do have a question about sexuality or a concern about something related to a disease you have been diagnosed with and treated for, you may need to be the one to open the door to a conversation with your health care provider. Don't wait till she has her hand on the door knob and is leaving the room. Start at the beginning, when you are asked why you are there that day. A statement like "I have a question about sex that I'd like to talk about" is clear and unambiguous. If the provider ignores you, leaves the room with a red face, or laughs, then you need another health care provider. Most will listen to your question and help you to find the answer.

And how do you talk to your sexual partner about sex? It should be easier than talking to a stranger, but usually it isn't. Most of us delay the conversation for days and weeks and months and years, and then it's really hard to talk about something after such a long time has passed. Many women have faked orgasms for many years, and so building the courage to finally admit that they haven't had an orgasm but have been pretending for all this time is really difficult. People can get defensive when they think that their sexual technique is being criticized. Telling the truth may hurt our partner's feelings, and no one likes to do that, so we keep quiet and no one is really satisfied.

Talking about sex with a third person in the room sometimes makes it easier. Consulting a sex therapist or sexuality counselor can help you and your partner talk in a meaningful way. The therapist or counselor is not going to watch you have sex (a common misperception about the work they do), is not going to make either of you undress (another myth), and is not going to ask you to tell secrets. The therapist or counselor will guide the conversation, be mindful of tension, and help you to avoid getting into a fight during the visit. This trained professional can help you to understand what is happening in your sexual relationship and why, and will be able to make suggestions to help you resolve long-standing issues.

CONCLUSION

Sexuality is a complex process that involves our brains and sexual organs. It is under the control of hormones but also involves established patterns of behaving and talking. Talking about sex is difficult, but if the brain is indeed the biggest sex organ, then we need to use our brains to formulate the words with which to talk to our sexual partner and health care provider when problems arise.

REFERENCE

World Health Organization [WHO]. (2004). Definition of sexual health. World Health Organization. Accessed December 31, 2008 from http://www.who.int/reproductive-health/gender/sexual_health.html#3.

SUGGESTED READING

General Sexuality

Barbach, L. *For Each Other*. New York: Penguin Books, 2001.
Brown, M., and S. Braveman. *CPR for Your Sex Life*. BookSurge.com, 2007.
Joannides, P. *Guide to Getting It On*. OR: Goofy Foot Press, 2006.

Women's Sexuality

Berman. J. R., and L. A. Berman. *For Women Only: A Revolutionary Guide to Overcoming Sexual Dysfunction and Reclaiming Your Sex Life*. New York: Henry Holt and Company, 2000.
Daniluk, J. *Women's Sexuality across the Lifespan*. New York: Guilford Press, 1998.
Ellison, C. *Women's Sexualities*. Oakland, CA: New Harbinger Publications, 2000.
Foley, S., S. A. Kope, and D. P. Sugrue. *Sex Matters for Women: A Complete Guide to Taking Care of Your Sexual Self*. New York: Guilford Press, 2002.
Hutcherson, H. *What Your Mother Never Told You about S-e-x*. New York: Perigee Books, 2003.
Klein, M., and R. Robbins. *Let Me Count the Ways: Discovering Great Sex without Intercourse*. New York: Penguin Putnam, 1998.
Leiblum, S., and J. Sachs. *Getting the Sex You Want: A Woman's Guide to Becoming Proud, Passionate, and Pleased in Bed*. New York: Crown, 2002.
Levine, S. B. *Sexuality in Mid-Life*. New York: Plenum Press, 1998.

Male Sexuality

McCarthy, B., and M. Metz. *Men's Sexual Health: Fitness for Satisfying Sex*. New York: Routledge, 2008.
Zilbergeld, B. *The New Male Sexuality*. New York: Bantam Books, 1999.

WEB SITES

http://sexuality.about.com/
This popular site for sexuality information provides balanced articles, tips, and conversations about sexuality.
http://www.goaskalice.columbia.edu/Cat6.html
This Web site is supported by the Health Services department at Columbia University. The Web site is set up in a Q & A format. It works to provide readers with reliable, accurate, accessible, culturally competent information and a range of thoughtful perspectives so that they can make responsible decisions concerning their health and well-being.
http://www.sexualhealth.com/
The Sexual Health Network provides access to sexuality information, education, mutual support, counseling, therapy, health care, products, and other resources for people with disabilities, illness, or natural changes throughout the life cycle and those who love them or care for them.

http://www.ourbodiesourselves.org/book/chapter.asp?id=13&gclid=CMfMr5Xtl5YCFQ
    OcFQodegkD6Q

Our Bodies Ourselves (OBOS), also known as the Boston Women's Health Book Collec-
    tive (BWHBC), is a nonprofit, public-interest women's health education, advocacy,
    and consulting organization. This is the group that wrote the landmark book, *Our
    Bodies Ourselves,* that educated multiple generations of women about their bodies.

http://nsrc.sfsu.edu/

The National Sexuality Resource Center (NSRC) gathers and disseminates the latest
    information and research on sexual health, education, and rights. NSRC initiates
    dialogues—both online and face-to-face—on sexuality to promote social justice and
    improve the quality of life in the United States.

http://www.siecus.org/

The Sexuality Information and Education Council of the United States provides resources
    to help educators, advocates, and parents provide accurate and appropriate informa-
    tion about sexuality to young people.

http://www.healthywomen.org/sexuality/index.html

The National Women's Health Resource Center operates this Web site, which provides
    information for women on various aspects of health and active living. The site has a
    large sexual health section.

http://www.indiana.edu/~kinsey/

The Kinsey Institute at Indiana University promotes interdisciplinary research and schol-
    arship in the fields of human sexuality, gender, and reproduction. The Web site has
    numerous links to other Web sites that take an academic approach to the study of
    human sexuality.

Part II

SEXUALITY AND ILLNESS

Chapter Three

SEXUALITY ACROSS THE LIFE SPAN

Sexuality is a lifelong process with particular milestones that occur during different phases and at different ages. This chapter highlights the important sexual milestones that are reached in each life stage, beginning with adolescence. Acute or chronic illness in any of these stages may impact on the achievement of these milestones and have far-reaching effects on personal growth.

PSYCHOSEXUAL DEVELOPMENT IN ADOLESCENCE

The hallmark of adolescence is the development of secondary sex characteristics that herald the change from childhood to adulthood. These physical changes in no way indicate that the adolescent has the maturity of an adult, but the adolescent's physical status may look like that of an adult.

In girls, the development of secondary sex characteristics usually occurs between the ages of 8 and 11. These developments have been taking place at younger ages over the decades and in some populations; for example, in African American girls, these developments may occur at even less than 8 years of age. The first change is the development of breast buds under the nipples. Soon after this, pubic hair begins to grow. This is followed by the growth of the internal reproductive organs (e.g., the uterus) as well as the labia (lips) of the vulva. By the 10th year, many girls will have their adult shape, with a defined waist and rounded breasts. They will have pubic and underarm hair and may have begun menstruation. Menstrual cycles are often irregular in the first year or two, but the girls are capable of becoming pregnant if they have intercourse.

Boys start maturing physically about a year later than girls. Starting somewhere around age nine at the earliest for most boys, the testicles enlarge and the skin of the scrotum thickens. The boy grows taller and develops muscles, and the shoulders broaden and the hips narrow. Underarm and chest hair appears. Genital growth continues with the appearance of pubic hair and the enlargement of the penis and scrotum. Many boys start to shave their facial hair, which has gradually changed from fine and fair to a somewhat coarser type. The voice also deepens in response to the larynx (voice box) growing larger. Most boys will have experienced a wet dream or nocturnal emission by the time they are 15. Many boys will have started to masturbate by this time too. By the end of puberty, most young men have almost reached their adult height, although men continue to grow into their twenties.

As well as being a time of physical growth and development, adolescence is a time when significant emotional and social changes occur. This is a time when peers are more important than parents, and during adolescence, the first stirrings of emotional attachment to members of the peer group occur. But many adolescents take longer to mature emotionally than they do physically, and while they may look like young adults, they still think like children. Most adolescents are preoccupied with how they look and constantly compare themselves to others in their peer group and images in the media. The comparisons are often unfavorable, and many adolescents suffer terribly because they think that they are not as attractive as their friends or the idealized pop stars they see on TV and in magazines. This may result in low self-esteem, and low self-esteem may lead to risky social and sexual behavior as teens seek to gain attention and popularity. Even though these adolescents look like adults, their cognitive thinking is more like that of children, and they are not able to think in the abstract or anticipate the consequences of many of their actions.

For adolescents who grow up in a loving and supportive family, where the parents are affectionate to each other and to their children, the passage to adulthood is usually achieved. Challenges remain, however; if the values in the home conflict with what the adolescent sees in his social surroundings, the adolescent will have to find a way to negotiate the dissonance between what happens at home and what happens outside the home.

The adolescent has some major tasks to complete by the end of this phase of development. He or she must separate from the family and achieve independence. The adolescent has to identify and then pursue a vocational goal. He has to achieve a mature level of sexuality and develop and maintain a realistic and positive self image. The adolescent also has to learn to control her impulses and deal with frustration, as well as learning to delay gratification of wishes.

During adolescence, sexual attractions usually occur; these may be attractions to members of the opposite sex or to members of the same sex. This can cause confusion for some adolescents, who are not sure who they are really attracted to and may feel pressure to self-identify as heterosexual, bisexual, or homosexual. Being something other than heterosexual presents a problem for many adolescents, as prevailing social attitudes denigrate homosexuals and adolescents are often desperately afraid of being different or other. Adolescents who are attracted to members of the same sex are often isolated and afraid and have few if any people to talk to about their feelings. This often leads them to engage in high-risk sexual behavior in an attempt to appear heterosexual.

The first sexual activity that most adolescents are involved in is masturbation. This is more frequent for boys than for girls and is usually a solitary activity. Some adolescents feel guilty about masturbating, as this activity still carries with it a sense of taboo, even though it is universally practiced even if not talked about! Because of the emphasis on safer sex and the risks associated with sexual intercourse, many adolescents perform mutual masturbation with partners, and oral sex is seen as an alternative to intercourse. This may cause some problems for parents, who may have a less laissez faire attitude to oral sex while their adolescent children see it as no big deal and not even as sexual activity.

Even though some adolescents are risk takers when it comes to sexual activity, when they are in a relationship, particularly one that is sexual, they place a great deal of importance on the emotional connection between them and their partners, and most adolescents want a sexually exclusive relationship. If one of them goes outside the relationship for sexual activity, the resultant pain and betrayal may be long lasting. Many adolescents lack the emotional skills to deal effectively with the breakup of a relationship, and this may lead to low self-esteem and self-worth.

Even though this age group is naturally curious and experimental, many young women become sexually active not because they really want to but because they think that everyone else is doing it and they feel pressured to conform. Some see this as the only way to get and keep a boy- or girlfriend. The fears and anxiety of their parents about the initiation of sexual activity are based on the idea that adolescents perceive themselves as immortal, invulnerable, and immune to the many consequences of risk-taking behaviors.

Most of the literature on adolescent sexuality focuses on the risks of pregnancy and sexually transmitted infections. There is little on teaching adolescents about healthy sexuality and sexual pleasure, which requires good communication skills and a sense of personal agency.

Adolescents generally use the media as information sources for their learning needs related to sexuality. Their peers are used to doing this, but their parents are not so used to it, especially if the parents are more conservative.

The depictions of sex that adolescents see in the media are focused on passion and pleasure and present sex in a positive light. This stands in stark contrast to their parents, who tend to focus on the negative aspects of sex, including pregnancy and infections, which they hope will frighten their children away from being sexually active.

When the Adolescent Is Ill

Illness during the adolescent years threatens the major lifestyle tasks of separating from parents and achieving independence, developing a positive self-image, and achieving a mature level of sexuality. Challenges to health, particularly if they are chronic, directly impact on the adolescent's ability to be independent and to separate from parents. The adolescent may need help with daily activities such as bathing, eating, and dressing. He may need help managing a complex regimen of medications and visits to medical appointments. Being away from school for extended or frequent periods of time distances the adolescent from her peers and marginalizes her in terms of the social activities of the peer group.

When treatments cause physical changes, the impact on body image and self-esteem cannot be underestimated. Imagine the adolescent with cancer who loses her hair during chemotherapy. She may be so embarrassed about this and feel so different and unattractive that she might refuse to return to school or go out with friends, because she knows that the other kids will be looking at her and judging her. The adolescent with kidney failure will also experience changes in the way his body looks. These patients are usually on large doses of medication that cause their faces to grow fat; this too can cause a great deal of unhappiness and make them feel that they are different and that their peers are laughing at them. Long absences from school interfere with normal social development, and some adolescents may find it difficult to interact with their peers if they have been away from the social group for a while. Serious illnesses and treatments may also impact on adolescents' ability to seek out romantic relationships, both because of appearance issues and because of a lack of self-confidence and a poor self-image. Some treatments interfere with normal growth and sexual development, so a 16-year-old may look more like a 10-year-old, with short stature and no secondary sexual characteristics.

Life-threatening illnesses like cancer fundamentally challenge adolescents' notion of themselves as immortal and invulnerable. Issues of mortality dominate much of the disease trajectory. Today over 80 percent of children and adolescents with cancer go on to become survivors, but their adult lives are affected both by the illness and by its treatments. Some patients are rendered infertile by chemotherapy or radiation; this may affect their decision to marry later in life. There is also the possibility that adolescents think they are infertile when in fact they are able either to conceive or to impregnate a woman, and if contraception is not used appropriately, unplanned pregnancy can result.

PSYCHOSEXUAL DEVELOPMENT IN YOUNG ADULTHOOD

While there is little change in the body of the person in young and middle adulthood (20 to 40 years), this is a time of tremendous emotional and social growth. This is the stage at which most people choose a mate and decide if they want children or not. Being diagnosed with an acute or chronic illness can disrupt plans and challenge individuals or couples in terms of the achievement of vocational and reproductive plans.

When the Young Adult Is Ill

The young adult who has a chronic illness faces a number of challenges to healthy sexual functioning. If not partnered at the time, he faces many challenges related to disclosure of the illness. When does one tell a potential partner that one has diabetes or has been treated for cancer? How do you tell someone that you have an ostomy bag or that you have scars on your body or a missing breast or testicle? How and when do you tell a potential life partner that you cannot conceive or will need fertility treatment in order to start a pregnancy? Is there a perfect time to disclose such significant information? How does one deal with the rejection that may follow such a disclosure?

Telling a potential partner soon after the first meeting is probably too early. One date does not mean that you are in a relationship, and telling the person then may be giving too much personal information too soon. If another date does not occur, you may be left wondering if it was the disclosure that ended things or if there was just no spark for the other person. But waiting for weeks may make it look as if you have been hiding the fact of your illness. It is difficult to decide on the best time to make your disclosure. Of course, there may be clues that you are dealing with a health issue; diabetics need to measure their blood sugar levels regularly and be careful with their diet, and some diabetics have to use insulin before meals.

Young adults with chronic illnesses often feel different from their peers and may not have reached the same developmental milestones as their disease-free peers. Think about young adults with leukemia. They may have spent an extended period of time having chemotherapy and may have missed a lot of time at college or university. They may find themselves isolated for extended periods of time when they are in hospital for treatment or dealing with the complications of treatment. They may miss many opportunities to meet potential partners through the usual channels. They may also be more dependent on their parents at a time when most young adults are making their own lives and have separated from their families. This dependence may be physical, in that they still live at home and may need help with some activities of daily living; they may be financially dependent as well, because they have not been able to find or participate in employment; and they may be emotionally dependent for these reasons too.

Fertility Issues

Fertility issues may affect both young men and young women after treatment for many chronic diseases; or a pregnancy may be too dangerous for some young women. Even though partners may have come to terms with this, they are often reminded by other people who ask, in a well-meaning way, whether they are planning to have children or by family members who pressure them, not knowing the facts.

In the crisis of diagnosis with a life-threatening illness such as cancer, many young people do not even think about future effects on fertility. If they were diagnosed as children or teenagers, their parents may not have considered this matter. Many people also assume that fertility treatments are more effective than they actually are. The most effective form of fertility treatment is sperm banking. A teenager or young adult man can produce sperm on two or three different occasions as little as 24 to 48 hours apart. The sperm are then frozen and can remain viable for many years. But there are challenges even with this relatively simple procedure. There are significant costs associated with sperm banking, and these are not usually covered by health insurance plans. A man may not have easy access to the laboratories and storage facilities needed, especially if he lives far from a major urban center. And this topic is often not discussed with the young patient for reasons including perceived lack of time, uncertainty about how to discuss it, and the acuteness of the illness, which may need immediate treatment precluding even a 48-hour wait during which to bank one or two samples.

The options for young women who must have treatment that affects the ovaries are much more limited. This is particularly challenging for the young woman who does not have a partner. Eggs do not freeze well, and even sections of the ovary are not able to survive an extended period of freezing. There is also the risk that some cancer cells may be present in the stored tissue and may survive the freezing and be reintroduced into the body when the ovarian tissue is reimplanted later. There is a great deal of research underway to solve some of these issues but at the present time, young women have few viable options unless they have a partner.

For the young woman who is partnered, the best option is to stimulate the ripening of multiple eggs with medication. These eggs are then harvested and mixed with the partner's sperm in the laboratory to create multiple embryos.

The embryos are then frozen and can be thawed and placed in the uterus of the woman months or years later when treatment is complete, or even in the uterus of a surrogate if the woman is not able to carry the fetus, for example in the case of a woman who has had her uterus removed. There are multiple ethical issues with this, however; if the woman does not survive or the relationship breaks down, what happens to the embryos?

PSYCHOSEXUAL CHALLENGES IN MID-ADULTHOOD

The years of middle adulthood range from 41 to 65 years of age. This is a time when most individuals are secure in their primary intimate relationship and have raised their children to young adulthood and independence. This is the time when many couples face retirement and is also the phase in which people are challenged by failing health and the onset of chronic disease. But this is also a time when some relationships fail or someone dies, and the challenges for the newly single remaining partner are significant.

During this time of life, some physiological changes in sexual functioning occur. For men, these changes usually involve the onset of some difficulties with erections, often associated with problems in cardiovascular health or diabetes. For women, starting in their mid-forties, perimenopausal changes start to occur, with the average age of cessation of menstrual periods at age 51. The decline in ovarian hormones leads to symptoms such as hot flashes and vaginal dryness, which both affect sexual functioning. Men and woman alike may find these changes difficult to accept and may fear that they are no longer sexually attractive to their partner. The messages in the media and in society in general are negative concerning the aging person, and middle-aged adults are often portrayed as being sexually unattractive and in need of plastic surgery, medications, hair dye, and makeup to appeal to others. If this message is internalized, it can have deleterious results for self-image and self-confidence.

This is amplified in the case of newly single middle-aged persons, who may not feel that they are capable of attracting someone new. But individuals in new relationships often find that their passion and sexual energy are rekindled with a new partner, and any difficulties related to treatment can be very frustrating. The strongest predictor of sexual health for midlife adults remains the presence of a loving partner who is interested in sexual activity; the poor health of the partner is the main reason why sexual activity ends.

PSYCHOSEXUAL CHALLENGES IN OLDER ADULTHOOD

For the adult over the age of 65, physical changes are inevitable. For many years, this has been a taboo subject, with the assumption that older couples are not interested in sex and are unable to have sex. The results of some recent studies turn those assumptions firmly on their heads. A survey of 4,000 men and women aged 64 to 65 years of age showed that, to the contrary, older couples are willing and able. These couples reported that they were satisfied emotionally and sexually by their partners, had intercourse on average twice a month, and found the sex enjoyable. The most important reason for a lack of sexual activity was that the partner had lost interest in sex.

In another large population-based study of adults aged 57 to 85 years of age, a gradual decline in the prevalence of sexual activity was seen, but with 53 percent of those aged 65 to 74 years and 26 percent of those older than 75 years reporting continued sexual activity. Women were less likely to report sexual activity as they grew older (perhaps related to illness and death in their male partners) and half of the respondents reported one bothersome sexual problem. For men this was erectile dysfunction and for women lack of desire, lack of vaginal lubrication, and problems achieving orgasm.

With increasing age comes the reality of physical changes and chronic disease. Diseases such as diabetes, cardiovascular disease, and arthritis all affect sexual functioning and are detailed in chapter 4 of this book. These conditions may cause sexual difficulties; the treatments, whether in the form of medication or surgery, can pose additional challenges. Antihypertensives prescribed to treat high blood pressure have a known effect on erections and ejaculation. Antidepressants affect libido and orgasm. Many of the medications used to treat heart disease have significant impacts on various aspects of sexual functioning. Despite this, many older adults continue to want and experience sexual activity well into the seventh and eighth decades of life. The basic needs we have for touch and affection are not reduced by age, and touch and affection may in fact become more meaningful with the years.

Elderly women often face the challenges of vaginal dryness with resultant pain during penetration. Other changes in the arousal phase include lessened swelling of the breasts; however, this usually does not pose a major problem. Weaker muscular contractions during orgasm may lessen sensation and alter satisfaction. Older men may have difficulty achieving and maintaining an erection, and the erection may be less firm than in earlier years. During orgasm, older men may produce less ejaculate, which may alter the sensation of orgasm. Older men may also notice that the refractory period, the time when a man cannot have another ejaculation, is lengthened and may persist for many hours or even days. Older adults also have to cope with reduced joint flexibility, which can make sexual positioning more challenging. They may also have reduced stamina and energy, which may dictate how vigorous sexual activity can be or dictate the frequency of sexual activity.

Older women report that as the years progress they are more interested in physical touch, kissing, and hearing loving words from their partner than they are in penetrative intercourse. This may be of some comfort to the older man who is having difficulties with erections. Older couples also report that the intimate connection grows deeper with the years and the relationship takes on a deeper spiritual quality than before.

One of the most challenging aspects of sexuality in the older population is a lack of recognition by health care providers that elderly people have sex, with the result that health care providers may not ask about this important aspect of quality of life when counseling the older adult about newly diagnosed conditions or prescribed medications. Many health care providers either assume that the elderly are not sexually active or are themselves embarrassed to talk about a topic with someone the same age as their parent or grandparent. This effectively leaves the older person or couple to raise the topic, and they may be just as embarrassed.

CONCLUSION

Illness at any stage of life may interrupt important psychosexual milestones. This has the potential to threaten various aspects of sexual functioning, including the establishment of sexual and romantic relationships, fertility, and sexual self-image.

SUGGESTED READING

Price, J. *Better Than I Ever Expected.* Emeryville, CA: Seal Press, 2006.

WEB SITES

http://www.siecus.org/
The Sexuality Information and Education Council of the United States is an organization that focuses on comprehensive sexuality education in the United States.
http://www.positive.org/Home/index.html
The Coalition for Positive Sexuality is another organization that provides honest sexuality education for teens.
http://www.plannedparenthood.org/health-topics/sexuality-4323.htm
Planned Parenthood promotes a commonsense approach to women's health and well-being, based on respect for each individual's right to make informed, independent decisions about sex, health, and family planning.
http://www.healthandage.com/
This Web site provides fact sheets on sex and aging for men and women.
http://www.apa.org/pi/aging/sexuality.html
This Web site is supported by the American Psychological Association. It is a resource for articles, books, and other sources of information on sex and aging.

Chapter Four

SEXUALITY IN MEDICAL DISEASE

Certain medical conditions have a direct effect on sexual functioning. These conditions are extremely common and occur across the life span but are particularly prevalent in adults of middle and older age. These conditions include heart disease, kidney disease, diabetes, arthritis, chronic lung disease, and multiple sclerosis. Even more common in today's society is obesity, which impacts on body image. Incontinence is another common complaint in women in midlife, and this has very real sexual effects. Sexuality is also impacted in people with HIV/AIDS.

CARDIAC DISEASE

David is 57 years old and a busy accountant in a large city on the West Coast. He's been married to his wife Marlene for 30 years, and they have two adult children who are married and live nearby.

David makes an appointment to see his internist because of something that has been happening over the last two months. For the first time in his life, he has been having problems getting an erection. Marlene tells him not to worry; she's 55 and going through menopause. But he is bothered.

He goes to his appointment pretty sure of the outcome. Dr. Fraser will give him some Viagra and all will be well. He's heard some of the guys at his office talking about this, and they all seem to be pretty pleased with their response to the little blue pill.

But Dr. Fraser doesn't just write the prescription; instead he sends David for some blood tests and tells him to make another appointment for the next week. David is a bit worried, but he's busy at work and forgets all about it until the day that he has to go back.

Dr. Fraser tells him that his cholesterol is high and his blood pressure is too high as well. He wants David to have some additional testing to see just exactly what is happening with his heart and blood vessels. David is shocked! All this from a problem with erections?

One in every three American adults suffers from one or more types of cardiovascular disease (CVD) in his or her lifetime, according to the American Heart Association (AHA). Due to advances in treatment, many individuals with cardiac disease are able and encouraged to maintain an active lifestyle, including sexual functioning, for the rest of their lives. Cardiovascular disease includes the following conditions: hypertension, coronary heart disease, angina pectoris, myocardial infarction (heart attack), acute coronary syndrome, hypertension (high blood pressure), and heart failure. Stroke and transient ischemic attacks are also caused by changes in the cardiovascular system. Disease in the blood vessels is caused by narrowing of the vessels, which causes a decreased blood supply to various organs. If the heart is affected, the person may have a heart attack. If the vessels to the brain are affected, a stroke may result. When the blood vessels in the penis are affected, erectile difficulties are the result.

Hypertension (high blood pressure) is a cause of erectile dysfunction (ED) in men, and some men may not take their prescribed medication to treat this condition, as the treatment may actually worsen their sexual difficulties. Women with hypertension also have sexual problems that are often ignored or not reported to health care providers. Individuals who have had a stroke experience global problems with sexual functioning, from loss of libido to alterations in orgasmic capacity. The psychological consequences are also important, with many stroke patients feeling sexually unattractive. Relationship distress and breakdown are not uncommon after a stroke, and altered sexuality may play a role in this.

While cardiac disease is often regarded as a disease of old age, many individuals with cardiac disease are actually younger; in fact, more than 50 percent of those with heart disease are younger than 65 years of age. In men, erectile dysfunction may be an early sign of cardiovascular disease, and it is important that any complaint of ED be followed up carefully with appropriate investigations. It is unclear whether or not sexual difficulties in women are also an early sign of cardiac disease; they may be, but there is insufficient evidence to reach a conclusion on this. The equivalent of ED in women is lack of vaginal lubrication; this is experienced by many women as a result of menopause and is also influenced by other factors such as their relationship with their partner, so a direct link to cardiovascular disease is more difficult to establish.

Three weeks later David is playing tennis with his old school friend. It's a hot day and the game is challenging. By the end of the second set, David feels sick to his stomach and tells his opponent that he has to take a break. His friend looks at him:

"You don't look too good, buddy. Maybe we'll just call it quits." David really doesn't feel well, and he agrees. He has a difficult time getting to his car; he feels weak and he's sweating buckets. He tells his friend that he doesn't think he should drive and the words are barely out of his mouth when he falls to the ground.

David is not aware of the next 45 minutes. An ambulance arrives and rushes him to the nearest hospital. He is seen very quickly and rushed off for an angiogram. His friend has called Marlene and she rushes to the hospital, only to wait three hours until some one can tell her what is happening and she can see her husband.

A young doctor eventually comes to see her. David has had a massive heart attack. The angiogram showed the blockage of two arteries supplying his heart muscle. The blockages were removed and he should recover fully. But he is going to need to make some significant changes to his lifestyle.

There are many myths about sexual functioning for those with cardiac disease. The most important and pervasive of these is the belief that sex is not advisable after a cardiac event such as a myocardial infarction (MI) or heart attack. The reality is that most patients can safely return to sexual activity following a cardiac event. Another misperception is that if a patient has heart disease, any sexual activity will lead to chest pain and potentially to a heart attack. But this is not inevitable. Perhaps the most egregious myth associated with cardiovascular disease is the idea that this is a disease of the elderly and that sex is no longer important to older adults. The error of this belief is shown in the responses of participants to the 1999 AARP/Modern Maturity Sexuality Study: approximately 67 percent of men and 57 percent of women considered a satisfying sexual relationship to be important to the quality of life.

But these myths do influence how the person with cardiac disease and his or her partner reestablish sexual activity after the diagnosis of a cardiac event. They also affect how health care providers perceive, treat, and educate these patients and their partners. This is important, because your health care provider may assume that because of your age you are not sexually active and may not give you important advice and guidance related to your condition. In addition, he may not think about sexual side effects when prescribing medications.

David is in the hospital for 24 hours and goes home feeling tired and sore. He has to have another appointment with the cardiologist in a couple of weeks, and he's told to take it easy till then. The hospital has given him some pamphlets to read about diet and exercise, and Marlene reads these from cover to cover.

Two weeks later, on a sleepy Saturday afternoon, David suggests that they make love. Marlene is a little shocked and more than a little reluctant. How safe is sex after everything he's been through?

So just how risky is sex? Certainly sexual activity affects heart rate and blood pressure. Masters and Johnson recognized this in their description of the human sexual response cycle (see chapter 2). In the excitement phase, heart rate, blood pressure, and respiration increase, and this could lead to greater fatigue in a person with advanced cardiovascular disease. These increases continue through the plateau phase, and just before orgasm, the heart rate may increase to between 110 and 180 beats per minute. After orgasm, heart rate, blood pressure, and respiration return to their normal levels.

Does sexual activity cause a heart attack? The risk from sexual activity is quite low. In a study of 858 patients who had experienced a heart attack approximately one week earlier, researchers found that sexual activity was a contributor in only 0.9 percent of cases. The relative risk of a heart attack in patients without a previous history of cardiac disease was similar to that in patients who had had a previous MI. The most likely time to have a heart attack is during the first two hours after intercourse. After cardiac rehabilitation (a special exercise and nutrition program), which is commonly prescribed for those who have had a heart attack, the risk of a patient who has already had a heart attack experiencing another heart attack due to sexual activity is only 20 in a million. People who are able to perform strenuous physical activity without chest pain will rarely experience chest pain (angina pectoris) during sexual activity; the risk is greater for their sedentary counterparts.

How much energy does sex require? In assessing the energy demands of sexual intercourse, we find that it has requirements similar to those of mild-to-moderate intensity exercise, for example, the equivalent of walking on a flat surface at a brisk pace (up to 5 km per hour), walking up two flights of stairs, driving a car, or talking about business. However, if the person is anxious or with a new partner, this may increase excitement and a greater increase in heart rate and blood pressure may occur, increasing the risk of an adverse event. The amount of effort required to have sex is also dependent on how strenuous the activity is and the position used by the couple. The man-on-top position uses the most energy for the man, and the woman-on-the bottom position is the least strenuous for the woman. Thus, changing who is on top can minimize cardiac effort for the person with heart health issues. Self-stimulation (masturbation) uses the least amount of effort.

> David accepts that Marlene is nervous about resuming their sex life. But he sees nothing wrong in getting back to life as normal. He's started to eat better and he goes for a long walk every day. He's already lost five pounds and is feeling better than he has for ages. Perhaps the medication that he was given for his blood pressure is helping too.
>
> One week later it's their wedding anniversary, and this time Marlene doesn't say no to David's invitation. But again he doesn't get an erection. He had a few glasses of wine with dinner, so perhaps that's it. But he's frustrated and getting a little angry with this body of his that won't do what he wants it to. The next morning he makes an appointment to see his internist. There must be something that can be done. He's only 57, after all!

It's not uncommon for a person with cardiac disease to experience sexual difficulties after a new diagnosis or hospital admission. Fear of a repeated cardiac event, fear of death, or fear on the part of the partner of causing an event can be a significant barrier to the resumption of sexual activity. New sexual difficulties may appear after a cardiac event; some men may experience an inability to have an erection, which is often associated with anxiety. Depression is also common after MI. It is also not uncommon for people to have difficulty finding ways to cope with cardiac disease, and some people become very distressed, which also leads to sexual dysfunction.

Medications used to treat cardiac disease may cause sexual difficulties for some people. Many of the medications used to treat cardiac disease (such as beta-blockers, angiotensin-converting enzyme (ACE) inhibitors, calcium channel blockers, and antihypertensives) may cause sexual difficulties. These include decreased interest in sex, problems getting or maintaining an erection, changes in ejaculation, decreased lubrication for women, or the inability to have orgasms for both men and women. Using alcohol in combination with these medications may increase the risk for sexual difficulties.

Treatment of Sexual Problems

Women who experience vaginal dryness due to any of the medications can use over-the-counter vaginal moisturizers (Replens) and lubricants (Astroglide or KY jelly) for sexual activity. If there are no other reasons why local estrogen treatment to the vagina cannot be used (a history of breast cancer, for example), then this is an effective option. There are no approved treatments for lack of libido in women, and problems with orgasm usually require specialized sex therapy and/or self-help books and videos.

The most common treatment for erectile dysfunction in men is one of the phosphodiesterase-5 (PDE5) inhibitors, such as sildenafil (Viagra), tadalafil (Cialis), and vardenafil (Levitra). These medications dilate blood vessels, which may lead to a dangerous drop in blood pressure in men with heart disease, and so the medications should be used with caution. Herbal or natural erectile medications that may contain sildenafil are not recommended. These medications should not be taken by men who are taking organic nitrates (nitroglycerin, isosorbide mononitrate, isosorbide dinitrate) and should also be used with caution in men with unstable cardiac disease and men with low blood pressure or significant heart failure. Men who occasionally use sublingual short-acting nitrates may still use PDE5 inhibitors under the direction of their physician but not within 24 hours of nitrate use. If you experience chest pain during sexual activity after taking a PDE5 inhibitor, you should call an ambulance. It is important to inform the emergency staff, including the ambulance attendants, that you have taken this medication, so that prompt and effective treatment can be given immediately. While there is no heart-related problem with using testosterone to increase libido in men, this hormone has been linked to the development of prostate cancer and so should be used with caution.

Resuming Sexual Activity

David sees his internist a few days later. Dr. Fraser has received the reports from the hospital and tells David that he's a lucky man. Things could have been much worse. David asks him again for some Viagra. Dr. Fraser sits down next to David and tells him that before he can even think of sex he needs to have some additional tests to make sure that it's safe to initiate sexual activity. And he tells David that he may not be able to take Viagra; it all depends on what medication he continues to take. David is surprised by this information. He had thought that everything would go back to normal.

It has traditionally been recommended that sex be avoided for six to eight weeks after a heart attack. In certain individuals, a satisfactory post-MI stress test sooner than six weeks after the attack allows sexual activity to be resumed after three to four weeks. However, in those who have suffered complications (hypotension, serious arrhythmia, or heart failure), sexual activity should be resumed more gradually, depending on the person's exercise tolerance (judged by a medically supervised stress test) and activity levels. By participating in a cardiac rehabilitation exercise program, people can increase their fitness and reduce the cardiac work associated with sexual activity. Exercise has also been shown to reduce the depression that often follows a heart attack and can also impact on sexual functioning.

Many people take longer to initiate sexual activity due to fear of complications or another cardiac event. The partner may be the one who is reluctant to engage in sexual activity due to fear. Couples should be advised to take as long as they need to resume an active sexual life, but they should share their thoughts about their needs and desires with each other. When sexual activity is resumed after a heart attack, couples should use any sexual position with which they are comfortable. But receptive anal intercourse is potentially dangerous for a person who has had a cardiac event, as stimulation of the vagus nerve in this position can cause an abnormally low heartbeat and decreased blood flow to the heart itself, which may lead to chest pain. Sexual activity should be avoided for three hours after a heavy meal, after excessive alcohol intake, in extreme temperatures, or when wearing restrictive clothing.

Two weeks later David has had a stress test and returns to see the cardiologist. His stress test was normal, his blood pressure is well controlled, and he hasn't had any chest pain or other complications. His weight is down even more and his cholesterol levels have responded well to the change in his diet and the medication. When asked if he has any questions, David blurts out, "What about sex? Can I try, doc?" Happily the answer is yes, and David tells the cardiologist about his problems with erections.

The doctor gives David some samples of Viagra and tells him to enjoy life but to continue with the lifestyle changes he has made. David goes home with a plan in mind and a smile on his face.

For those couples who choose not to resume having sexual intercourse, alternatives to intercourse are both normal and acceptable. Nonpenetrative activities (such as oral sex or mutual masturbation) provide sexual pleasure and satisfaction without the fear that intercourse may be harmful. Some couples find that the kissing and touching that usually comprises foreplay can be satisfying and an end in itself.

If you do experience chest pain and you have nitroglycerin on hand, you should take the prescribed amount and notify your physician if the pain is not relieved within 15 minutes. You should also report any shortness of breath, dizziness, persistent increase in heart rate or blood pressure, and extreme fatigue following sexual activity.

MULTIPLE SCLEROSIS

Sylvia is 35 years old and a librarian at a small community college. Two years ago she met and married one of the professors at the college. She'd never expected to get married and had hardly dated in her teens and twenties. Meeting Robert was an unexpected blessing and they have a lovely life together. One year ago, Sylvia fell in the garden for no apparent reason. And not just once: she fell twice in the same day. She was also really tired and found herself going to bed at 9 p.m. most nights. Robert was concerned about this and urged her to seek medical attention.

She saw her physician a week later. He did some tests and called her back with the news: she had multiple sclerosis (MS). Sylvia was not as upset as Robert; she had a sister with MS who lived a full and busy life with three children and a demanding job as a museum curator. But Sylvia's disease took on a much more debilitating form than her sister's, and she quickly developed other signs of the disease. One of the first things she noticed, besides the fatigue, was changes in her sex life. This bothered her a lot, because having discovered sex relatively late in life, she really enjoyed it! It started with some numbness in her genital area and soon she started having difficulty having an orgasm.

Robert was understanding and told her repeatedly that sex was not that important. But she was upset by these changes and this is what really depressed her.

Multiple sclerosis (MS) is a progressive disease affecting the central nervous system that is often diagnosed in people between the ages of 20 and 40 years. Because there are different types of MS, some people have relatively few problems while others can be severely affected quite quickly. This disease affects all aspects of daily life, including sexual functioning. Physical functioning is altered due to changes in muscle strength, problems with bladder and bowel functioning, and altered sensation. Psychologically, people with MS may notice increased emotional instability and also depression. One of the major impacts of MS is on the energy level of the individual with the disease, and fatigue is an integral part of the disease experience for most individuals.

All of these factors may lead to sexual difficulties, which are reported by up to 85 percent of those with MS. The most commonly reported sexual symptoms are altered genital sensations, lack of vaginal lubrication, difficulty achieving orgasm, and loss of desire for sex in women. Men most commonly report difficulty achieving and maintaining an erection and ejaculatory problems. Common to both men and women are leg spasms and spasticity, which can interfere with sexual activity, fear of urinary and fecal incontinence, the passing of flatus during sexual activity, and fear of embarrassment related to this. Issues related to body image and feelings of attractiveness, or lack of attractiveness, are also experienced, mostly by women.

> Sylvia's form of MS seemed to gallop along. Within a year she had difficulty walking and had to use a walker outside the house. She had taken an extended period of sick leave and tried to go back to work half time, but she was just too exhausted and her balance problems made it difficult for her to do her job properly. So she went on long-term disability leave, which almost broke her heart. She loved her job and the people she worked with, but most of all, she loved the students. Now she spent most of her days reading. It took her so long now to do any of her usual tasks in the house. Robert did all the shopping and chores; he seemed quite happy to do this but she felt useless and sad.

Fatigue is experienced by up to 95 percent of those with active MS. In part this is caused by challenges in coping with activities of daily living and the expenditure of energy in fulfilling social and family roles. In addition, people with MS also expend a large amount of energy coping with heat in the environment. Muscle spasticity also uses a large amount of energy, and most people with MS find that they need to nap during the day. Exhaustion at night also precludes energy for sexual activity at the end of the day. Solutions to this include finding time during the day when energy levels are at their highest to spend time with one's intimate partner. Some people use stimulants such as caffeine to increase their energy, but this often has the effect of irritating the bladder and causing bladder spasms or incontinence. A physical therapist or occupational therapist can suggest strategies to minimize energy expenditure and maximize physical function. Alternative positions for sexual intercourse that reduce energy use can also help. The person with MS may find it easier to be on the bottom or in a side-lying position for intercourse. Finding activities other than intercourse may also be helpful; oral sex may provide as much if not more sexual stimulation without requiring a large amount of energy.

Depression is common among people with MS; up to 50 percent have experienced one or more major depressive episodes. Depression may occur as a result of MS lesions in the brain or as a reaction to the multiple challenges faced by the individual and the many losses that go along with this disease. Many of the medications commonly prescribed for the treatment of depression have sexual side effects that exacerbate the challenges to healthy sexuality already experienced. These include difficulties with arousal and orgasm.

People with MS also experience *nerve pain,* most commonly burning, tingling, or numbness of various parts of the body. Very often these occur in the legs and perineal area (the vulva for women, and between the scrotum and anus in men). The effects on sexual activity are obvious. Some people also experience pain in the area around the mouth, which makes kissing and oral sex painful. Living with chronic pain also contributes to the fatigue mentioned above. Finding medication to treat nerve pain can be frustrating; as with all medications, the side effects may have unintended effects on sexual functioning. Many of these medications cause sleepiness, which may lead to a lack of interest in sex or an inability to stay awake during sexual activity, and this can be stressful for the partner! Nonmedicinal therapies have been shown to be helpful in the treatment of nerve pain. These include acupressure and acupuncture, massage therapy, and biofeedback. Some people also respond well to the application of hot and cold packs to the affected area two to three times a day.

> Sylvia managed to get through each day, but barely. She so looked forward to seeing Robert at the end of the day, but increasingly she felt that they were no longer man and wife but rather patient and caregiver. He had to help her with so much these days. She needed help getting out of bed, and she no longer bathed because getting into and out of the tub was both painful and embarrassing. He'd bought a special stool for the shower, and she used that with him just outside the door in case she needed help.
>
> She had a lot of pain too but kept this hidden from her husband. Her doctor knew about it and had given her a prescription for a stronger painkiller, but Sylvia was reluctant to take it. Just this past week a new symptom had popped up; she'd had some really painful muscle spasms when she was lying in bed. She wasn't sure that Robert had noticed, but it seemed that her whole left leg had risen off the bed. It had happened again the next morning while she was waiting for Robert to help her get dressed. And she'd had an accident, right there in the bed! She was so embarrassed about this. She didn't tell Robert and she covered up the wet spot on the sheet. It had taken her all morning to change the sheets and do the laundry. Robert was really surprised when he came home and saw that she'd washed the sheets, because he always did this. But she couldn't tell him why she'd had to do it.

Individuals with MS also experience *sudden muscle spasms* that are both painful and distracting when the individuals are involved in sexual activity. Sometimes a limb extends or flexes for no apparent reason, or the limb may not relax, causing cramping and pain. Spasticity can also interfere with the ability to find a position for sexual intercourse that is comfortable or optimizes sexual pleasure. Pharmaceutical treatments for spasticity usually involve some combination of muscle relaxants and antiseizure medications that often contribute to fatigue, so finding a balance between relief of symptoms and prevention of further side effects is a delicate matter. Taking medication about 20 minutes before sexual activity maximizes the good effects of the medication before the sedating side effects occur. Physical therapy can be helpful in exercising limbs and maintaining flexibility. For sexual activity, the couple may need some help finding positions that allow for sexual pleasure but minimize spasms or spasticity. For the man who experiences spasms or pain when he is in the man-on-top or missionary position, any position that allows him not to place weight on his legs may be helpful. These include the female-on-top or side-lying positions. For the woman who experiences lower limb problems, the side-lying position may help, as will placing her legs over her partner's pelvic area while lying on her back. This position means that the two people will not be facing each other, but it also allows for more ready access by either partner to the woman's clitoris, which may be stimulated effectively by hand or with a vibrator.

Bladder and bowel problems are also common in MS. Incontinence (not being able to control the bladder), needing to pass urine often (called frequency), and urgency (feeling an urgent need to empty the bladder) are the most common effects on the urinary system. All of these can impact on sexual functioning, and the fear of having an accident during sexual activity, or actually experiencing one, can cause avoidance of sexual activity. Other people find that they are not able to empty their bladder completely and so have a sensation of pressure, which interferes with pleasurable sexual sensations. Some people have to catheterize themselves to empty their bladder; timing this before sexual activity can help in alleviating symptoms of pressure and can also reduce fear of leakage. For those with an indwelling catheter, sexual intercourse is possible, but care must be taken to avoid disturbing the catheter, which lies in the urethra. For men, wearing a condom prevents the catheter from moving too much; the catheter should be placed backward along the length of the penis, with the condom covering the penis and catheter. Women should tape the catheter to the groin area, and care should be taken in the insertion of the penis into the vagina that traction is not applied to the catheter. There are medications available to treat overactivity of the bladder, but these too have side effects. Lifestyle changes such as limiting both intake of fluids and type of fluids can be helpful. Caffeine and alcohol both irritate the bladder, and soft drinks containing aspartame as well as caffeine are known to cause frequency and urgency and incidents of incontinence.

For those who have difficulties passing feces or find that constipation is an issue making intercourse uncomfortable, judicious use of laxatives or manual removal of feces before intercourse may be helpful. Emptying the bowel before sexual activity reduces the risk of accidents and embarrassment, but laxative use may increase the risk of some leakage of soft stool or even diarrhea.

Sylvia still mourned the loss of their sex life. They still cuddled before going to sleep, and once or twice a month they tried to have intercourse. What really happened is that Sylvia tried and Robert went through the motions to please her, but she could see that his heart wasn't in it. She wanted to ask him why but was afraid that he'd lie to her. She couldn't bear that. But she was also afraid that he'd tell her the truth. What if he found her unattractive? What if he couldn't even think of her in that way anymore?

The direct impact of MS on sexual functioning is caused by brain and spinal cord lesions. These most commonly result in reduced sensation in the genitals and problems with arousal (lubrication in women and erections in men) and orgasm for both men and women. Men with MS may find any one of the PDE5 inhibitors (Viagra, Cialis, or Levitra) helpful in achieving and maintaining an erection. Women may find that a vaginal moisturizer such as Replens can help with vaginal dryness. For sexual intercourse, a water-, glycerine-, or silicone-based lubricant is more effective. Vaginal estrogen is the most effective treatment for vaginal dryness, but women may not want to take additional hormones or they may not be advisable.

For many women with MS, a major factor in their ability to be interested or active sexually is the way that their body image has been affected. Some women maintain a positive body image and see themselves as attractive and desirable. Others find that their view of themselves is negative and are challenged to even think of themselves as sexually attractive even to their long-term partners. This can cause relationship distress and even the breakdown of some relationships.

Despite all the suggestions made above, the most important factor underlying sexual relationships is the ability to communicate one's wants, needs, desires, and feelings. Some couples find it easy to talk about these issues while others struggle. Seeking professional help from a couples or marital therapist can help to encourage open communication about the challenges not only of sexuality in the context of MS but also of the role changes and threats to the marital relationship posed by this chronic, debilitating disease. A sexuality counselor or therapist can also provide suggestions specific to sexual problems.

ARTHRITIS

Stan is a handsome 66-year-old man who lost his wife to cancer 10 years ago. He has one adult daughter, who has encouraged him to find someone for some time now. She can see how lonely he is, and he really doesn't get out much. He loves to spend time with her two children, but they are not suitable companions for a man his age.

And besides, they're entering their teen years and won't want to hang out with their granddad for much longer.

Stan loves to dance, and he starts going to the local community center, which holds a dance for singles every Thursday night. The first couple of times he went were really difficult; they just reminded him of how much he missed Elsie, his wife. But there was a nice crowd at the center, and he soon started chatting to a group of men who mostly sat around talking and did very little dancing. They encouraged him to ask one of the ladies to dance, and he did, and soon they were swooping and swirling around the floor and getting quite a bit of attention from the rest of the dancers. All that activity played havoc with his knees, but it felt so good that he just took extra medication for the pain and kept on dancing.

That first dance set up Stan for many more. He was an accomplished dancer, and the ladies were all after him. But there was one who caught his eye; Patti was short, with dark hair and green eyes. He'd danced with her that first evening, and the smell of her perfume lingered on his clothes. Three weeks later, he mustered the courage to ask her to go for coffee and then for dinner, and now they were a pair and the rest of the dancing ladies went into mourning.

The best-known forms of arthritis are osteo- and rheumatoid arthritis. However, there are in reality 120 different kinds of arthritis, including Sjogren's syndrome, fibromyalgia, and gout. Osteoarthritis and rheumatoid arthritis are perhaps best known, and their effect on sexuality is easier to understand because there is greater understanding of the physical manifestations of these conditions than of some of the rarer forms.

Rheumatoid arthritis (RA) is a chronic, progressive, inflammatory disease that affects the joints. Osteoarthritis (OA) is a degenerative disease that destroys the cartilage in the joints with the growth of bony spurs that cause pain and stiffness. The end result is often an individual with chronic pain, fatigue, and depression, all of which impact on sexual functioning. Deformity of the joints may result, and this is frequently seen in the fingers of those affected. The hip and knee are also commonly involved in OA, and with the increase in the population of adults over the age of 55 years (the baby boomers), this has become a widespread problem. Two-thirds of people with OA experience sexual problems related to their disease.

The first time Stan and Patti planned to make love was scary for them both. Stan hadn't been with anyone other than his wife, and because of her cancer, they hadn't had sex for three years before she died. Patti had never been married; she had lived with a man for about 10 years but that was long ago.

But attraction and the beginnings of love give one all sorts of courage, and they were both eager to move their relationship to the next level. Stan was not sure that everything would work as it should. He knew that things changed as you got older, and he'd sure noticed that he didn't have erections so often anymore. But Patti made him more excited than he'd been for many years, and he just hoped for the best.

And when it finally happened, it wasn't his penis that let him down. That worked just fine. It was his knees! The pain was awful and he thought he might even have let out a yelp of pain. Patti was understanding and even made a joke about it, but he didn't think it was that funny. In fact, he was pretty embarrassed and wasn't sure he wanted to try again.

The level of sexual problems seen in people with RA is even higher; 85 percent of women and 69 percent of men state that joint pain and swelling play a part in the decision whether or not to initiate sex with a partner. Both the hips and knees are joints that are used actively during sexual intercourse in men and women; the man-on-top or woman-on-top positions place pressure on both hips and knees. This may cause avoidance of sexual activity due to fear of pain, or it may decrease sexual pleasure, which in turn can lead to a lack of interest.

Sexual problems may be compounded by medications. A common treatment for inflammation is steroids, and these cause alterations to physical appearance with extended use. The typical results of extended use of steroids are a bloated face, thin arms and legs, and a hump on the back between the shoulders (buffalo hump). Changes to the body can significantly alter one's self-image as a sexual being, and these changes can alter one's feelings of attractiveness. In addition, steroids cause loss of interest in sex, depression, and sometimes mania. Long-term use of these medications can also result in skin rashes, ulcers in the stomach and mouth, and hair loss.

At times it is the partners' concern about causing pain for the person with OA or RA that causes the problem; partners may avoid sexual touching and activity or try to get it over with as quickly as possible, depriving themselves and their partner of sexual pleasure and satisfaction. This can lead to feelings of rejection and distress and even marital breakdown. For the person who lives with the constant daily pain of OA or RA, the experience of pain in association with sexual activity often leads to anticipation of pain, which leads to avoidance. Partners may feel guilty that their needs are the source of pain and suffering.

Stan and Patti continue to see each other, but the issue of sex is like the elephant in the room. They don't talk about it, but they think about it a lot. They kiss and cuddle and still enjoy dancing, but that's not all there is to a relationship. Stan has to see his primary care provider for a new prescription of his pain medication. Jane is a nurse practitioner, and she is really easy to talk to, so, when he sees her, he tells her about his problem.

Even though she's hardly older than his daughter, Jane is very professional and doesn't seem in the slightest bit shocked. She even has some literature for Stan to read from the Arthritis Society. She tells him that he might find some useful information in there, and she also gives him a Web site address that has even more information. Stan's not sure about this; he hardly uses the computer and he can't ask one of the grandkids to help him this time! Jane also suggests that now might be the time to consider having one or both knees replaced.

Addressing the concerns of the person with arthritis is important for the couple, so that realistic plans can be made, either to make sexual activity more comfortable or to look for alternatives to intercourse. Strategies for increasing comfort include taking pain medication shortly before initiating sexual activity, taking a warm bath or shower to relax muscles, placing pillows and other supports carefully to protect joints, using sexual positions that minimize pressure and pain, and using alternatives to penetrative intercourse such as mutual masturbation with or without the use of vibrators or oral sex. As with all other conditions affecting sexuality, the ability to achieve clear communication about what works and what causes pain is important.

SJOGREN'S SYNDROME

Sandy is 56 years old and a homemaker and mother who dotes on her family. She has never worked outside the home and loves to garden, do craftwork, and bake. She has always volunteered at her son's school and for his hockey team.

Sandy went through menopause beginning at 50. She had all the symptoms: hot flashes, weight gain, mood swings and irritability, and horrible, heavy periods. Her doctor suggested that she take hormones but Sandy wasn't interested and toughed it out.

Six years later most of those symptoms are gone. She no longer has her periods and she only has the odd hot flash in the summer months. She's much less irritable now and is glad of that. There were times back then when she thought she was going to go crazy! But she has one last problem that just won't go away: her vagina is really dry and painful. She hasn't let Barry her husband touch her down there for five years now. She thinks that it's part of the menopause, but when she tells her family doctor this, he asks some additional questions and sends her for some blood tests. He calls her the next week with some news: she has an autoimmune disease that she's never heard of.

Although not well known, Sjogren's syndrome affects almost 4 million Americans, 90 percent of whom are female. It is also more common in older women. Sjogren's is a chronic autoimmune disorder that affects the moisture-producing glands of the body. This produces dry eyes and mouth, and particularly a dry vagina, which in turn causes pain during intercourse. The symptoms of this disease develop slowly over about 10 years and often start at the time of menopause. The stress of having a chronic illness also reduces vaginal moisture, and one of the frustrations of this disease is that it often goes undiagnosed for many months and women are told that their symptoms are related to menopause.

Solutions

Treatment includes strategies to help reduce or control vaginal dryness. Local vaginal estrogen is very helpful, and oral hormone therapy containing estrogen will help most women. But many women are reluctant to take estrogen due to concerns about its effect on the breast and heart. There are also reports that oral estrogen lowers the quality of life and well-being in women with Sjogren's syndrome. Vaginal moisturizers such as Replens, a polycarbophil that clings to the vaginal walls and releases moisture into the lining of the vagina, can be very helpful in maintaining comfort for the woman every day but are not useful for sexual activity. To have an effect in reducing pain during intercourse, a lubricant is necessary; some of the more useful lubricants are either silicone or glycerin based. When intercourse is painful, women tense up in anticipation of the pain, and a cycle of tension, muscle spasm, and pain is set up. This can be difficult to treat, so prevention is better. The woman needs to find ways to relax during sexual activity. This may mean that penetration is avoided for some weeks to allow her to become comfortable with other forms of sexual touch that do not include penetration. Outercourse (where the penis is placed between the lubricated upper thighs of the woman and thrusting is initiated) can be helpful to both partners. Limiting the time of penetration can also help, as most women with this disease cannot tolerate long periods of friction even if there is no initial pain with penetration.

LUNG DISEASE

Jim is 55 years old and looks years older. He's not had an easy life; he grew up poor and stayed poor. He's worked as a farmhand most of his life, but since his lungs started giving him trouble, he's mostly stayed home while his wife works at the grocery store in their small town.

Jim has smoked two packs of cigarettes a day since he was 10 or 11 years old. His dad smoked and his brothers too, and no one told them it was bad. And they lived into their seventies. Except for his one brother, who fell off the barn one summer and broke his neck.

Jim manages to live with the results of his smoking. He coughs a lot, and in the morning he may cough for 20 minutes or more when he first gets up. He has trouble catching his breath most of the time, too. So he just sits as quietly as he can, because moving around makes him short of breath. It's a horrible feeling, and sometimes at night he wakes up in a cold sweat trying to get some air into his lungs. He sometimes wonders if he'd have started smoking all those years ago if he had known what life would be like now....

Chronic obstructive pulmonary disease (COPD) is extremely common, affecting up to 16 million Americans. It is caused by smoking predominately, although some people may develop this condition due to exposure to environmental irritants. A central experience of the person with COPD is that of shortness of breath, which is not only experienced as a physical symptom but has emotional consequences as well. Many people with COPD will over the years develop fatigue related to the constant fighting for breath, wheezing, and coughing. The constant effort to breathe also causes weight loss due to the expenditure of large amounts of energy just to breathe.

While there is almost no evidence on what happens to women with COPD, we know that men with COPD are more likely to experience erectile difficulties than their healthy counterparts in the population. The reason for this may in part be physiological, with changes to the tissues of the penis due to inflammatory processes. But a major contributory factor is the use of medications to treat COPD that tend to cause erectile dysfunction. Living with a chronic debilitating condition can also affect sexual desire.

Solutions

Some strategies to address this include the use of PDE5 inhibitors for men with ED, unless the man is on nitrates for the management of chest pain (angina). Changing medications may also help, if the sexual changes result from the use of specific drugs. If shortness of breath occurs with the effort of sexual activity, changing positions so that the affected person has to make the least effort may be helpful. Side lying or placing the affected person on the bottom is generally suggested to be effective. As with many other conditions where fatigue is a contributing factor, oral sex or mutual masturbation can provide sexual pleasure with less energy expenditure. Using a short-acting bronchodilator before sexual activity may also help to open airways and make breathing easier.

DIABETES

Ken has been a diabetic since he was 13 years old. The diagnosis was a huge shock to his parents, but he pretty much ignored it. He tried to do what his mom told him to, but it wasn't easy to be the odd one out all the time. It was really difficult keeping to the diet, and some of his friends made fun of the lunch he brought to school in a brown bag. They all ate at the fast-food place across the road from school, and Ken often just threw his lunch from home in the garbage and ate fries and burgers with the rest of the guys.

He's now 24 years old and for the last two years he's been really careful about controlling the glucose levels in his blood. Even though he had lots of teaching about diabetes when he was younger, it was too difficult to follow the recommendations, but now he's better at it. He sees his doctor regularly and checks his blood glucose levels three or four times a day. He's even stopped drinking. Most of this is because of Jenny.

He's been dating Jenny for three years. They both go to the same church and are looking forward to getting married when she finishes her teaching degree next summer. They have decided to wait until they're married to have sex. She wants to do this more than he does, but he goes along with the idea. It's really hard to do this; he loves her so much and it just seems to be the natural thing to do. A part of him is a little worried about that, though. He's not sure that everything's working the way it should. There are times when they're fooling around and he doesn't get hard. That shouldn't happen to a guy his age, should it?

Diabetes is an extremely common disease affecting many millions of Americans. Diabetes causes problems in many body systems, including the cardiovascular system, the kidneys, and the nervous system. Diabetes has been linked to the epidemic of obesity in North America and is an insidious disease, some times labeled "the silent killer," as the damage to organs occurs over time and many with the disease are diagnosed only when significant damage has been done.

It is well known that men with diabetes experience erectile problems, but less is known about women with diabetes. The erectile response in men is in part vascular, as blood fills the spongy tissue of the penis, and in part neurological, as this filling is dependent in part on messages from the nerves supplying the penis. It should be easy to see how nerve and blood vessel damage would then result in erectile difficulties. The same vascular influences occur in women: women with diabetes report decreased lubrication (alterations to blood supply to the vaginal tissue result in less lubrication), which is an important factor in sexual arousal. A lack of lubrication tends to cause pain during intercourse, which then lessens the desire for sex in order to avoid the pain. About 50 percent of people with diabetes will experience neuropathy as a result of their diabetes. This can cause pain, tingling, and numbness of the hands and feet, which can interfere with sexual pleasure and desire. The skin is also a large erogenous zone, and the altered sensations can be a powerful challenge to engaging in sexual activity.

Women with diabetes, particularly Type 2 (or adult onset) diabetes, also have higher levels of androgens, which may affect sexual functioning in a negative way. Women with poor control of their blood glucose levels also have more frequent urinary tract infections, and these can cause irritation of the vulva and pain during sex.

Depression is also common among people with diabetes, and the effects of depression on sexual functioning result in sexual problems; these may then be compounded by treatment with SSRIs such as Paxil or Prozac that cause problems with desire and orgasm. People with diabetes often gain weight, and the associated body image changes may negatively impact on sexual self-concept. The high blood glucose levels experienced by diabetics with poor control negatively effect energy and mood. Irritability does not encourage feelings of well-being in the diabetic or her partner and may be a further challenge for the couple.

Solutions

So what can be done about this? Early diagnosis of diabetes is important, and tight control of blood glucose levels may help to minimize organ damage that can affect sexuality. Exercise will not only help to control levels of glucose in the blood but it can also help alleviate depression and control weight, both of which are known to affect body image and sexuality. Just like a physical workout, sex can impact on blood glucose levels, and some diabetics may find that they need to have a snack handy if their glucose levels fall during or after sex. For those people who have an insulin pump, it can be left on during sexual activity or removed completely; alternatively, the tubing only can be removed and the infusion set left in place as long as it is well anchored. Stopping the infusion for up to an hour is probably safe, but each person should be aware of the signs of high blood glucose and prepare to restart the pump immediately after sex.

The treatments for arousal difficulties are the same as for anyone who has problems in this area. Oral medications for erectile dysfunction are useful unless there are other medical conditions that preclude the use of these medications. The vacuum pump and penile injections also work for those who cannot take the pills or don't respond to them. For women, vaginal moisturizers and lubricants can be effective in treating vaginal dryness. Caution should be used with glycerin-based lubricants, which may increase yeast infections. It may take longer for both men and women with diabetes to become aroused.

Extra time should be spent kissing, touching, and actively stimulating the penis and scrotum in men and the clitoris in women. This may be tiring for both the person with diabetes and the partner. Using a vibrator can really help with this, and the extra stimulation from the vibrations may be very pleasurable even without intercourse.

HIV/AIDS

John and Judy, a couple in their late thirties, are both addicted to drugs and alcohol. They are also both HIV infected and have known about this for almost three years. They live in a house that they share officially with two other people, but unofficially there are about eight people living under the same roof. Life is a struggle for John and Judy; they try to make ends meet by working odd jobs and in the summer they usually find work with a traveling carnival. But it's hard.

They receive their medical care at a clinic at the county hospital. They get their HIV treatment free and they are very grateful for this; they both know that without it, they'd probably be dead. They've also been in and out of drug rehab programs over the years. It's hard to remain clean and sober when everyone around is taking some form of alcohol or drugs.

Recently they've both noticed something weird going on with their sex life. Both of them are having problems; she's numb down there and he's having problems getting hard. Judy wants to ask their nurse at the clinic about it, but John is not keen; they were given a hard time by the staff when they first started going there. The staff was insisting that they needed to use condoms with each other, but John didn't see the point. They were both HIV positive, so how could condoms help? He's not sure that the staff is going to be interested in their sexual problems.

HIV infection, and the resultant immune deficiency syndrome called AIDS, was once a death sentence for those affected. Over the years, with the development of effective treatments including highly active antiretroviral therapy (HAART), infected individuals may expect to live with a chronic infection and a better quality of life than in the early years of the epidemic.

In the early years of the epidemic, the topic of sexuality in HIV/AIDS concerned safer sex and the prevention of the sexual transmission of the virus. As people now live longer, attention has moved to the quality of life of those living with HIV/AIDS, and some interesting observations have emerged. Both men and women are experiencing sexual problems, especially if they are using a combination therapy that includes a protease inhibitor. This drug regimen is extremely common, and so potentially many people taking these drugs will experience problems. For men, erectile dysfunction appears to be a real issue. This may in part be due to HIV damaging the nerves responsible for erections, although this is likely to happen in men with more advanced disease. A contributing factor to this may be the effect that HAART has on lipid levels and the resultant development of cardiovascular disease, which is known to affect erections. Men with more advanced HIV infection also have lowered testosterone levels, but the ED occurs even in men who are not showing any signs or symptoms of disease, and when men stop taking the protease inhibitors, their ED resolves. The use of nucleoside reverse transcriptase inhibitors (NRTIs) leads to alterations in genital sensation that may also contribute to ED.

For women with HIV/AIDS, multiple stressors are likely involved in sexual dysfunction, although the research on women is scant. Women may experience a lack of sexual desire in response to the diagnosis of HIV infection, and this may result in avoidance of sexual activity in part related to a fear of transmitting the infection to a sexual partner. For some women, this may impact negatively on their ability to continue in a relationship. This in turn may lead to depression and the use of alcohol and recreational drugs, all of which contribute to a decreased quality of life and increased risk of risky behavior.

Women also appear to suffer from treatment-related side effects affecting sexuality. NRTIs contribute to altered sensation in the genital area, and numbing can lead to sexual avoidance or a lack of interest if sexual pleasure is affected. Despite this, many women with HIV continue to be sexually active after diagnosis, and fear of abandonment by a partner may mean that a woman continues sexual activity with him, even though she has no interest or does not experience sexual enjoyment or satisfaction. Women with HIV/AIDS are also more susceptible to a variety of sexually transmitted infections (STIs) including human papilloma virus (HPV), which causes genital warts and trichomonas, a vaginal infection. Vaginal yeast infections (candida) are also more common and difficult to treat. All of these will cause pain with penetration.

For both men and women, a significant side effect of HAART is the development of lipodystrophy. This syndrome includes weight gain in the abdominal area, a fat pad between the shoulders (buffalo hump), and loss of fat under the skin of the legs, arms, and face. This syndrome is highly recognizable, particularly in the gay community, and effectively labels one as HIV infected. Body image has always been an important factor in the social and sexual lives of gay men; these tell-tale signs of disease impact not only on self-image and sexual image but also on the ability to attract potential partners and are a visible stigma and a threat to many. Given that women in society today experience many of the same anxieties related to body image, women with HIV infection will also experience a stigma and threats to the integrity of body image similar to those of gay men.

People with HIV/AIDS frequently don't tell their health care provider that they are having sexual problems. There has always been tremendous pressure on those infected with HIV to be sexually responsible, limit their sexual partners, and use condoms or latex barriers during all sexual acts. Admitting to having difficulty maintaining an erection with a condom may be too fear provoking for a gay man. The inevitable next question will likely be: "Are you having sex without a condom?" and the ensuing lecture about safer sex may not be what the man wants or needs. So the actual extent of sexual problems in the gay population is probably underestimated.

Solutions

A careful assessment of drugs used, both prescribed and recreational, is important in identifying possible causes of sexual dysfunction. Men with more advanced disease may have low testosterone, which can be corrected with supplementation and careful monitoring for the development of prostate cancer. Medications such as megestrol and ketoconazole also lower testosterone levels.

The PDE5 inhibitors (Viagra, Cialis and Levitra) must be used with caution in men with HIV/AIDS. Viagra and Cialis should be taken with care by men who are also taking protease inhibitors, NRTIs, ketoconazole, itraconazole, and erythromycin; lower doses of the PDE5 inhibitors should be taken, always under the supervision of a qualified health care provider. These drugs should not be used if you are taking ritinavir. Taking poppers to increase sexual pleasure is also dangerous if you are taking a PDE5 inhibitor. The vacuum pump, penile injection, and the intraurethral pellet (MUSE) are effective treatments for ED and are likely safer given the cautions referred to above.

Women should report any episodes of pelvic pain or pain during intercourse. Screening for STIs and prompt treatment may alleviate any pain. For HIV-infected women who experience early menopause and the associated symptoms of vaginal dryness, hormone therapy with close monitoring may be warranted. The use of vaginal moisturizers and lubricants can also help, although care should be taken *never* to use oil-based lubricants as these destroy the latex in condoms and dental dams and allow the transmission of HIV and other organisms.

RENAL DISEASE

Mark is a young man who has struggled with kidney problems since he was a teen. He's getting married next year to a lovely woman he met at the dialysis clinic. She had an infection when she was younger and her kidneys failed. Last year she had a transplant and is doing really well. She says she hates the way she looks; the drugs that she takes to prevent rejection of her new kidney make her face look fat, but Mark loves her just the same.

Mark is waiting for a kidney. He was adopted as a baby and so he doesn't have any blood relatives who could donate a kidney to him. So he just waits and waits. He's used to the dialysis and he's formed friendships with some of the nurses who work there. And that's how he met Pam, his fiancée.

Pam wants to wait till they're married to have sex. And he's okay with that, because he's really not that interested in sex. He knows that's strange for a guy his age, but maybe it has something to do with his kidneys or something. He'd like to talk about it but he's not sure who to ask.

Kidney disease is a significant problem in North America, with millions of people affected. Individuals with kidney disease experience a range of threats to the quality of life, including problems with sexual functioning.

Individuals with chronic kidney disease (CKD) report alterations in sexual desire, arousal, and orgasm. This is more common among patients on dialysis; 60 percent of men undergoing this kind of treatment report a lack of desire and absence of sexual fantasies. This may be corrected by having a kidney transplant; men who have been transplanted report that their libido returns very soon after the surgery. Erectile dysfunction is also common among men with kidney disease, with almost half of men reporting problems with erections.

Women on dialysis have even more problems with libido, with almost 100 percent reporting a lack of desire. This improves after transplantation but not to the same extent as in men. Women also report problems with arousal disorder, with many reporting failure to experience lubrication and pleasurable sensations. Among adults who were treated when they were children, many report a lack of satisfaction in their sex lives as adults. As with many other chronic diseases, fatigue plays a large role in sexual functioning, and repeated visits for dialysis add an extra layer of exhaustion.

Chronic kidney failure also causes changes in reproductive hormones and in another hormone, prolactin, which is linked to libido. Depression and low self-esteem are common in the population suffering from chronic kidney failure, and these factors may play a role as well as the emotional difficulties caused by living with this condition. Many people with kidney disease also have high blood pressure, and the antihypertensive medications used to treat this are known to affect erectile functioning in men as well as genital arousal in women.

Chronic kidney disease also causes alterations in body image. Obesity is common, and for those on dialysis, the scarring from the sites where the needles go in can cause embarrassment. For those with advanced disease, changes in skin tone due to an accumulation of toxins are common. In addition, weight loss may occur and limbs may swell. Those who have a kidney transplant report an improvement in sexual interest but have ongoing issues with body image. The drugs used to prevent rejection cause weight gain, growth of body and facial hair, and acne.

Solutions

Erectile functioning can be improved with the use of the PDE5 inhibitors; these appear to be safe in men with renal disease or after kidney transplantation unless the men are also on nitrates for chest pain. Other erectile aids such as the intraurethral pellet (MUSE), the vacuum pump, and penile injection are also effective after appropriate education and counseling. Penile implants are not recommended for men who have had a transplant, as the antirejection medications will cause rejection of the implant.

Treatments for women with low libido and decreased arousal are often difficult to find. Counseling for the woman and her partner may help; suggestions for alternatives to sexual intercourse and adapting to fatigue can be useful. Counseling can also help women who are experiencing body image concerns. But perhaps the best that can be done is for women to learn to adapt and accept the changes.

INCONTINENCE

Wendy has a problem, just like her mother and grandmother before her. She pees in her pants. It's that simple and that bad. Ever since she had her three kids, who are now between the ages of 12 and 16, she's had this problem. It happens when she sneezes or coughs or laughs. And forget about going to the gym! That would just be a nightmare. But the worst part is that she leaks when she and George, her husband of 20 years, have sex.

She can't avoid sex, although she'd like to. So she makes sure that she takes a shower before sex, and once George is done, she gets up and has a good wash down there. George is always complaining that she lacks spontaneity; why does she always have to shower before sex? It breaks the mood for him, but she just won't stop.

Incontinence, the involuntary loss of urine, is fairly common among women and increases with age. The two most common kinds of incontinence are stress incontinence, in which loss of urine occurs with sneezing, coughing, or exertion; and urge incontinence, in which the loss of urine occurs after a sensation of urgency but the one follows the other very quickly and the woman does not have sufficient time to get to the toilet. Both forms of incontinence are associated with sexual problems.

For women who experience incontinence, great efforts are made to conceal this fact (by using pads and sprays or frequent washing to minimize odor) or to control it (by frequent visits to the restroom or avoidance of physical exercise). Some women avoid social situations in which they are not sure of their access to a restroom. But when sexual activity is affected, the usual response is to avoid sex, which in turn leads to relationship distress.

Up to 60 percent of women with stress incontinence experience leakage during sexual activity. This leakage is more likely to occur with penetration, in contrast to women with urge incontinence, who tend to experience leakage with orgasm. But the consequences of this go far further than what happens in the bedroom. Women who suffer from incontinence often lose the desire for sex. This is in part due to embarrassment but also due to the fact that the leakage of urine at all times alters the environment of the vagina and often leads to painful intercourse. When aroused, many women find it difficult to relax and will often go to the bathroom multiple times during foreplay to ensure that their bladder is empty and to preempt involuntary leakage. Fear of leakage also leads to problems with orgasm; knowing that orgasm will cause leakage, many women do not relax and in fact hurry their partner to finish; this in turn can cause problems for the partner, who may develop premature ejaculation due to the pressure to get it over with. Women go to great lengths to cover up their incontinence by taking frequent showers, having intercourse in the shower or bath only to mask any leakage, using feminine sprays to mask odor, or padding the bed with sheets or towels. While some of these coping mechanisms are effective, actually seeking help is ultimately more sensible.

Male incontinence is less common and may be a side effect of surgery on the prostate or urethra. When involuntary leakage occurs during sexual activity, often during arousal or orgasm, it may cause the same consequences for the man, with embarrassment and avoidance of sexual activity or even erectile dysfunction due to fear of further leakage.

Fecal incontinence, the involuntary loss of feces or stool, is another condition that causes great shame, perhaps even more so than urinary incontinence. Sexual avoidance is very common, and surgical treatment seems to offer little relief. Perhaps the patterns of avoidance set up before surgery continue, despite improvements in symptoms.

Solutions

There are a number of treatments for incontinence that, if successful, will also treat the sexual dysfunction associated with it. There are oral medications that are effective in treating urge incontinence. Many of these have side effects, but there are different types that can be tried and a consultation with a physician can be the first step.

Pelvic floor physiotherapy, where the muscles of the pelvic floor are strengthened through exercises, has been shown to be effective both in controlling leakage and also in improving sexual functioning. Both men and women see improvements after learning and doing the prescribed exercises. Electrical stimulation of the muscles of the pelvic floor is also helpful although slightly more invasive. For those who are not helped by medication or exercise, surgery is usually the next step, and there are various options for both men and women

A major challenge in the treatment of incontinence is that many people with this condition are reluctant to seek help. This may in part be due to embarrassment or to acceptance of incontinence as a part of aging.

OBESITY

Jenny has always been heavy; her grandmother said she had a glandular problem and to make her feel better gave her cookies. Her grandmother's been dead for 18 years, but Jenny has continued to eat those cookies and anything else sweet and soft. Jenny is now a large woman in her early forties. She lives alone and works in the accounts department of a department store. She has some friends at work, and they go out to eat every Friday at noon. Their favorite place to eat is a diner across the road from the store where the club sandwiches are four inches thick and the fries are the best in town. Most of the girls are married, and they tease Jenny about finding a man. But who would want her? Jenny knows that no man would even give her a second glance. Everyone tells her she has a lovely face, but that face is as round as the moon and the body underneath it is as soft and puffy as the Michelin man. No one is going to want her in that way, that she knows for sure.

Obesity has been associated with sexual dysfunction in different ways. Obese individuals are more likely to feel unattractive, experience less enjoyment from sexual activity, and have more difficulty with the performance of sexual acts, and they are also likely to avoid sexual activity. Obese men are also more likely to have erectile dysfunction than their normal-weight counterparts, but obese women are more affected by poor body image, lowered desire for sex, and avoidance of sexual encounters.

Much of the research on obesity and sexual difficulties has been done on individuals who have had gastric bypass surgery for morbid obesity due to their need to lose a substantial portion of their body weight. Less is known about those who are only slightly or moderately overweight. Given that people who are overweight often have a negative body image, and that we know that body image has an impact on sexual self-concept and confidence as well as on the desire for sex, it is perhaps not unreasonable to believe that even moderate obesity can affect sexual functioning. Obesity is often linked to cardiovascular disease, which is linked to erectile dysfunction in men.

Solutions

Lifestyle changes such as diet and exercise are the cornerstones of treatment of mild to moderate obesity. Loss of weight should equate to improved self-image and increased sexual confidence, but evidence in the scientific literature is lacking. There is, however, strong evidence for improvements in sexual functioning among the morbidly obese who lose significant amounts of weight following gastric bypass surgery.

CONCLUSION

This chapter has described the many sexual problems experienced by people with medical conditions. While there is a physiological basis for many of these problems, the psychological component cannot be ignored. Many people with chronic ill health have a negative view of themselves, and this affects sexual functioning. These issues often go ignored in their encounters with health care providers, and unless chronically ill persons ask about these issues, the problems may not be addressed as part of routine care.

WEB SITES

Cardiovascular Health

http://www.womenshealthmatters.ca/centres/cardio/index.html
This Web site is produced by Women's College Hospital in Toronto, Canada. The site provides evidence-based information for women that is approved by the medical staff at the hospital. Each health topic is supported by resources and information related to the diagnosis and treatment of the condition.
http://www.americanheart.org/presenter.jhtml?identifier=1200000
This comprehensive Web site contains information from the American Heart Association. All aspects of cardiac health and disease are covered, and there are videos, information sheets, and opportunities to post questions on this interactive Web site.
http://www.cdc.gov/DHDSP/
This is the website of the Centers for Disease Control and Prevention and their Division for Heart Disease and Stroke Prevention. There are links on this page to various policy reports, statistics, and Web sites that provide information for people with heart disease and for those who want to prevent it.

Respiratory Health

http://lungdiseases.about.com/od/generalinformation1/Respiratory_Health_Lung_Diseases.htm
This is a section of the popular About.com Web site. It provides user-friendly information on various kinds of lung diseases.
http://www.medicinenet.com/lungs/focus.htm

MedicineNet.com is an online health care media publishing company. It provides easy-to-read medical information for consumers on a user-friendly, interactive Web site. The page on lung disease describes a long list of conditions that can affect the lungs.

Diabetes

http://www.diabetes.org/home.jsp
This is the Web site of the American Diabetes Association. It contains information for consumers and health care professionals as well as the latest news on diabetes, recipes, and tips for healthy living.
http://befitoverfifty.com/pages/diabetes.htm?source=GooAds
This is another Web site dedicated to providing information on diabetes, but this one focuses on people over the age of 50.

Multiple Sclerosis

http://www.mssociety.ca/en/pdf/sexuality.pdf
This is a link to a document that provides detailed and comprehensive information about multiple sclerosis and sexuality.

Renal Disease

http://www.kidney.org/atoz/atozItem.cfm?id=108
The URL provided is for the Web site of the National Kidney Foundation. The link provided is to a page that contains information specifically about kidney disease and sexuality.

Arthritis

http://arthritis.about.com/cs/sex/a/sexualityarth.htm
This is a section of the popular About.com website. This Web site provides information about arthritis and sexuality, with links to other Web sites.

HIV/AIDS

http://hivinsite.ucsf.edu/insite?page=pb-daily-sex
This Web site from the University of Southern California, San Francisco, provides useful information for people living with HIV/AIDS about safer sex and disclosure to sexual partners.

Incontinence

http://www.continence.org.au/site/index.cfm?display=112772
This is a section of a Web site provided by the Continence Foundation of Australia. It contains suggestions for managing incontinence during sexual activity as well as a question and answer section.

Chapter Five

SEXUALITY IN SURGICAL DISEASE

Some surgeries, such as hysterectomy, have the potential to cause alteration in sexual functioning. Others, such as heart surgery, may precipitate a fear of sexual activity. People who have an ostomy in which all or part of their colon is surgically removed also have special needs related to altered sexual functioning. Orthopedic surgery often has a positive effect on sexual functioning as it alleviates the pain of damaged joints. Men who develop an enlarged prostate may need surgery that has a very real impact on sexual functioning even though it alleviates the bothersome urinary symptoms. This chapter will highlight some strategies to deal with common issues in the preoperative, perioperative and postoperative periods, including limited joint mobility, body image issues as a result of scarring, and pain that interferes with normal sexual functioning.

HYSTERECTOMY

Rita started having heavy periods in her late forties; she knew this was the start of menopause but she didn't expect it that it would start this early or that it would be so bad. It was really bad. Every time she got her period, and these now came closer together, she had to stop all her usual activities. She bled and bled and even started passing clots as big as salad plates. She felt tired most of the time, and her friends commented that she didn't look well. So she went to see her primary care provider; this provider sent her to a gynecologist, who told her she had fibroids and her uterus needed to come out. And that had to happen soon.

Hysterectomy is the second most frequent surgery performed on women of all ages. The only surgery performed more frequently is cesarean section. Forty percent of women will have had a hysterectomy by age 64 years. During the surgery, the uterus is removed and often the uterine tubes and ovaries are removed at the same time; this is called an oophorectomy. The surgery may either remove the cervix or leave it in place. This surgery may be performed via an incision in the abdomen; it can also be done using newer laparoscopic techniques, in which four or five small incisions are made in the abdominal wall rather than one larger incision. The surgery can also be done internally, with the uterus being removed via the vagina. Among premenopausal women, this surgery is most often performed because of severe bleeding, often associated with fibroids or with hormonal changes during the menopausal transition. Among postmenopausal women, the surgery is often performed for the correction of prolapse of the uterus and bladder in the pelvis. A minority of women have this surgery because cancer is present in the uterus itself, the cervix, or the ovaries.

Effect on Sexual Functioning

Rita had the surgery three weeks after she saw the gynecologist. Her recovery went well, and within about two months she was feeling almost like her old self. Her husband Joe hadn't been sure that surgery was necessary (all the women in his family just waited it out), but he's changed his mind. Rita seems so much more energetic and she's even seemed interested in resuming their sex life, which, when he thinks about it, had pretty much died off in the past year or so.

Historically, little attention has been paid to the role of the reproductive organs (the uterus, uterine tubes, and ovaries) in sexual functioning. It was thought that these organs had little to do with libido and sexual pleasure. Any changes that occurred were thought to be of a psychological nature (it's all in your head) rather than having a physiological basis. A lack of understanding of the changes resulting from the removal of these organs formed the basis for negating the effects of hysterectomy on sexual functioning or for the erroneous belief that all women would show the same symptoms following the surgery. It is now understood that different women will experience different changes and that these changes are real and based not in their heads but rather in the anatomical and physiological changes resulting from the removal of these organs.

Early studies of the effects of hysterectomy on sexual functioning showed some contradictory findings. Women were noted as experiencing less interest in sex following the surgery, irrespective of whether the ovaries were removed or not. But other studies suggested that women experienced an increased interest in sex when the uterus was removed and some even experienced greater sexual satisfaction. It's important to remember that women who are having problems with bleeding or pain, common reasons for having this surgery, are usually not having sex often. The bleeding and the pain interfere with normal sexual activity. It follows then that when the source of the problem is removed, a woman's sexual life may improve too. If the uterus is removed because there is cancer there, the result may be slightly different, as she then has to have further treatments and the prospect of cancer is very different from that of having a hysterectomy to control heavy bleeding or pain.

When the cervix is removed during the surgery, nerves and blood vessels supplying the pelvis are destroyed or damaged. These nerves and blood vessels are contained in a structure called the uterovaginal plexus. Many experts think that the nerve and blood vessel damage causes ongoing problems for the woman sexually. The upper third of the vagina is known to enlarge during arousal, and damage to the nerves may impact on this, potentially causing pain for the woman with penetration. Nerve damage may also alter the amount of lubrication produced during arousal.

Removal of the cervix may also result in the vagina being shorter; this can cause pain with penetration. Scar tissue may also develop at the top of the vagina where the cervix used to be, and this scar tissue may also cause pain with penetration. It has been suggested that preserving the cervix (in a sub-total hysterectomy) would minimize sexual problems after hysterectomy, but this practice has not gained great favor among gynecologists. The rationale for removing the cervix is that this prevents cervical cancer, but regular Pap smears essentially take care of that problem.

The cervix is also a source of lubrication and if it is removed, lubrication is decreased; this can also cause pain for the woman. Other women find that the cervix is a trigger for orgasm; when the penis bumps against it during thrusting, orgasm occurs. Absence of the cervix may therefore interfere with the occurrence of orgasms.

The uterus itself moves during orgasm, and many women describe this sensation as being an integral part of the pleasure of orgasm. When that organ is absent, some of the pleasurable sensation is lost. But, conversely, removal of the uterus permanently removes the risk of pregnancy, and so for some women, hysterectomy may in fact be sexually freeing as the risk of pregnancy is permanently removed. The absence of a uterus also means that menstruation will not occur, and for some women, this may also result in greater sexual freedom and enjoyment.

Studies have also shown that some women experience feelings of emptiness and depression following removal of the uterus. For women who regard their reproductive status as an important part of the way they see themselves as women, the absence of the uterus may result in negative feelings when the uterus is removed. Some women may also experience alterations in body image with the presence of a scar on the abdomen. If the ovaries are removed from a premenopausal woman, the resulting symptoms of rapid onset menopause, often more exaggerated than in normal menopause, may also influence her experience.

Removal of the ovaries, particularly for the premenopausal woman, results in an immediate absence of the ovarian hormones, particularly estrogen. This will result in extreme symptoms of menopause including loss of vaginal lubrication. Many women report that a surgical menopause is very difficult, and when compared to natural menopause, the symptoms do seem to be much worse.

There are also problems with the way most of the research on this topic has been carried out. Many of the studies do not use validated questionnaires, and they use measures of sexual functioning that do not reflect the reality of women's sexual lives. For example, frequency of sexual activity is related to the presence of a partner who is willing and able to have sex. Women can have sex even if they don't want to or feel little desire. Women are enrolled in these studies just before their surgery, a time when their symptoms are at their worst and their sexual lives impacted by these symptoms. Thus, improvements after the surgery may be exaggerated. Overall, however, studies suggest that hysterectomy results in no change or some improvement in the sexual lives of the women who have this surgery.

COLON SURGERY

Debbie has had Crohn's disease since her late teens. She's had to learn to cope with the pain and the bloating, and for the past 15 years, the medication has helped a lot. She got married last year to Bill and they hope one day to have children. Soon after they returned from their honeymoon, Debbie noticed that the medication just wasn't helping. She was having frequent bouts of diarrhea and the pain was getting much worse. She saw her gastroenterologist, who suggested that perhaps it was time to consider surgery.

Individuals with Crohn's disease or ulcerative colitis, two forms of inflammatory bowel disease, frequently need to have surgery when oral medications no longer control their symptoms. Surgery for Crohn's disease usually involves the removal of parts of the bowel; depending on which parts of the bowel are removed, individuals may need to have a temporary or even a permanent ostomy. This surgically created diversion allows wastes to be collected in a bag through a stoma on the abdominal wall.

For those with ulcerative colitis, the entire bowel and rectum usually need to be removed. In the past, individuals would have a permanent ostomy, but today a more common surgery is the creation of a pouch inside the body that acts as the rectum and collects stool. This is called an ileoanal pouch. With this pouch, you can pass stool normally but you will have many loose movements each day as the colon, which usually extracts water from stool, is no longer there. For those who enjoy anal sex, surgical removal of the rectum can present a unique challenge.

Sexual functioning is affected in people with Crohn's disease and ulcerative colitis. In women with Crohn's, sexual activity is limited because of abdominal pain, diarrhea, and fear of losing stool involuntarily. These women also complain of pain during intercourse. Women with ulcerative colitis also complain of vaginal dryness, which causes painful intercourse, and have similar fears about leakage of stool during sexual activity. Men with these conditions do not appear to have any sexual problems until they have surgery.

How Does the Creation of a Stoma Affect Sexuality?

Debbie was really nervous about the surgery, even though she knew it would help alleviate her symptoms. Bill just wanted her to get well. She knew that she would have an ostomy following the surgery, but she was not prepared for how she felt about it when she saw if for the first time. It looked so red and raw and she just burst into tears. The nurse who was with her tried to comfort her, but all Debbie could think was that her life was ruined. Everything was ruined. How could she have children after this? How could she and Bill ever make love? It was disgusting; *she* was disgusting. It was all ruined.

For both men and women, living with an ostomy creates significant body image issues. Both the ostomy itself and the bag used to collect the feces can elicit feelings of distress. People with an ostomy may react with shock and disgust soon after surgery, and they often say that they feel sexually unattractive. An additional issue is the way their sexual partner(s) will react to the ostomy and bag. Some partners may react negatively to the ostomy, while others are cautious in their response; of course, some will be positive. Both the individual with the ostomy and the partner may be concerned about what it looks like and may also fear damaging the ostomy or causing pain to the person during sexual activity. The person with the ostomy may also be concerned about odor, leakage, gas, or noises emitted from the bag.

The stoma on the skin (where the bowel opens onto the skin) always looks red and moist, and touching it often causes a little bit of bleeding, which can cause anxiety for the person and the partner. The emotional and psychological aspects of living with an ostomy and bag are real: some people with an ostomy say that they feel baby-like and that much of their life is focused on keeping clean, changing the bag, and making sure that it does not leak. Having an ostomy means that something that is usually very private is now much more visible. For some, this will conflict with an adult sense of self and self-control, and this may cause problems in intimate relationships.

Following surgery to create an ileoanal pouch, men may experience difficulties with erections as well as problems with ejaculation. Some men do not have any ejaculation with orgasm; this may be because the tube that carries sperm to the prostate (the vas deferens) is cut during the surgery or because the ejaculate flows back toward the bladder instead of to the outside (retrograde ejaculation). Men may notice a difference in the sensation of orgasm when ejaculate does not flow though the penis.

What Can Be Done about This?

Depending on the nature of the sexual problem, there are a number of different strategies to address the issues. Men who have erectile difficulties can try one of the oral agents such as Viagra, Cialis, or Levitra unless they have specific contraindications to these medications.

If these do not work, a man may want to try the vacuum pump, or the pellet that goes into the urethra (MUSE). Injections into the body of the penis are usually the next step and, finally, a permanent surgical implant may be inserted. Retrograde ejaculation is usually not a major problem unless fertility is still desired by the couple. An explanation of why retrograde ejaculation occurs is usually enough for men who do not want to father more children. If fertility is an issue, there are ways to extract the sperm from the urine, and referral to a fertility specialist is a good idea.

For women, painful intercourse may be alleviated by trying positions other than the man-on-top for penetrative intercourse. With the woman on top, the depth of thrusting can be controlled by her. The side-by-side position can also help with this. Some women prefer to avoid penetrative intercourse altogether; alternatives such as oral sex and mutual or solitary masturbation may be satisfying to both partners. Another alternative is outercourse, in which the man places his erect, well-lubricated penis between the thighs of the female partner and initiates thrusting in that position.

On the afternoon before Debbie was being discharged from the hospital, a young woman came to see her. This young woman was a volunteer with the Ostomy Society and she had an overstuffed bag over her shoulder. She introduced herself as Linda and told Debbie her story. She too had Crohn's disease, she had also had surgery, and she had lived with a stoma for five years. She had gotten married the previous year and showed Debbie the photos of her wedding that she had stored on her cell phone. Debbie was amazed that here was a young woman, very much like her, who seemed to be coping so well. Could that happen to her too with time?

Linda opened the large bag that she carried. Inside it were all sorts of pieces of fabric that she explained to Debbie. They were things that Linda had used over the previous five years to help her deal with having an ostomy and a bag. With a twinkle in her eyes, she pulled something else out of the bag. "The Ostomy Society doesn't know that I show these to people . . . but they saved my sex life." She showed Debbie a pair of lacy panties with a slit in the crotch . . . Debbie wasn't sure what they were for, but she was sure that Linda was going to tell her!

If you have an ostomy, there are a number of things that can be done to increase your comfort with the bag. You may find that using a belt or cummerbund to stabilize the bag can help to reduce fears that the bag will become disconnected from the stoma. Emptying the bag just before sexual activity can also reduce anxiety. If you or your partner is disturbed by the sight of feces in the bag, an opaque cover over the bag can be helpful. Some people are able to use a cap that is placed over the stoma during sex, which allows greater freedom as the bag is not there at all. Using a smaller bag during sex can also help, as this is less bulky than the usual bag. Women may want to try crotchless panties; these conceal and anchor the ostomy and bag but allow the genitals to be easily accessible for foreplay or intercourse. Wearing clothing to hide the bag can also increase confidence and make a woman feel better. A teddy or peignoir may make a woman feel more attractive, but a comfortable T-shirt or men's cotton shirt is a cheaper and some say sexier alternative. For men, wearing boxer shorts stabilizes the bag, and the opening allows access to the genitals.

If fear of odor is a concern, having a bath or shower before sexual activity and using perfumes, colognes, or deodorizers can also be helpful. Another strategy is to avoid foods and drinks that cause gas or odor; this may also help to prevent leakage or inflation of the bag.

Trying different positions for sexual intercourse can also help to prevent pressure or weight on the abdomen. The woman-on-top position and the side-lying position can be very successful, especially if the person lies with the stoma on the side closest to the surface. This allows the bag to fall away toward the surface and not come between the partners. The rear-entry position, either kneeling or lying, in which the person with the ostomy lies in front of the partner, also prevents pressure on the bag. But these positions may pose some challenges for people whose mobility is impaired or for those with other disabilities.

CARDIAC SURGERY

Bob and Elsie are in their late sixties, and recently they moved to Florida from their home in Ohio. They love the warm winters and are both active in their retirement community. Six months before moving to Florida, Bob had a quadruple bypass graft. His doctor told him he was lucky to be alive, because the blockages in the four vessels were almost completely cutting off the blood supply to his heart muscle. Bob made a good recovery from the surgery. Since moving, he has been more physically active than he was previously and is feeling better than he has for many years.

They've made some close friends in the community in the few months since they moved. Elsie in particular has a group of female friends, all about the same age.

They laugh and joke about all sorts of things, including their husbands. The other women joke about sex all the time; Elsie's not sure that Bob would be happy to know that this is what they talk about. Since his heart surgery, they haven't had sex and haven't talked about it either. Elsie thought that the doctors probably told Bob that he couldn't have sex any more and he just didn't want to talk about it. That was fine with her. But she's not sure that Bob is all that happy about it.

Not much is known about sexual functioning after cardiac surgery, including coronary artery bypass graft (CABG) or heart transplantation. Because many of those requiring these surgeries are older and because of the severity of the conditions leading up to these surgeries, perhaps it has not been considered important to do research in this area. But it is clear that individuals having these surgeries do think that information about sexuality is important, and health care providers are urged to give information to all patients having this surgery.

From the few studies that have been done, it appears that both men and women fare equally in terms of sexuality after cardiac surgery. This is not necessarily good; while both men and women reported that in the six months after CABG, sexual functioning had gradually resumed, there were significant challenges. Two-thirds reported that their level of activity was the same as in the six months before surgery, a time when they were likely to have felt sick and when sexual activity was limited by their physical condition. Almost one-third stated that they were less sexually active in the six months following the surgery. It takes quite some time for the sternum (breast bone) to heal after it has been cut during the surgery. Breathing, moving, coughing, and so forth are all affected by how well the sternum has healed. Once the sternum has healed properly, the individual who has had the surgery will feel much better and may be more willing to think about sexual activity. Heart transplant recipients are known to have global sexual difficulties including decreased frequency of sexual activity, erectile and ejaculatory problems, and difficulty having orgasms.

Some of the problems may be caused by the multitude of medications that most people who have had cardiac surgery continue to take. But the problems, particularly lack of sexual activity, may also relate to a lack of information about sexuality and an assumption by people who have had cardiac surgery that they are lucky to be alive and should not bother to ask about sex or even have sex. They may also assume that sexual activity places an undue burden on the heart. The same cautions that apply to individuals who have had a heart attack apply here: if you can manage moderate exercise, then you can safely have sexual intercourse. The same modifications also apply: the person who has had cardiac surgery may want to be more passive or the couple may want to avoid intercourse and instead engage in mutual masturbation or oral sex.

ORTHOPEDIC SURGERY

People with arthritis in their knees and hips often experience pain during sexual activity. This is detailed in chapter 4. The hips and knees are especially important during sexual intercourse due to the fact that the most common position for intercourse, with the man on top, places a great deal of pressure on the man's knees in particular and his hips to a lesser degree. If the woman is the one with arthritis, it is also easy to see how her hips and knees might be affected if she is on the bottom during sex. The medications taken for pain relief may also have an impact on sexual functioning.

Surgery in the form of hip and knee replacement is increasingly being offered to those who have serious arthritis. The surgery is usually successful and allows people to regain quality of life, mobility, and exercise tolerance. It also allows some couples to resume sexual activity where previously it was just too painful. There are a limited number of studies on this topic: however, there is good evidence that joint or hip replacement allows people to become more active and that their chronic pain resolves.

BENIGN PROSTATIC HYPERTROPHY

Art is 63 years old and a professor at the university. He teaches history and is known among the students as someone who genuinely cares about them and their learning. But lately he has had less patience with his students, his colleagues, and his wife. Beth is his wife and she's noticed that he gets up a lot at night to pass urine. This disturbs her sleep so she counts how many times he gets up; this past month it's been 8 to 10 times a night. No wonder he's grouchy! The poor man hasn't had a decent night's sleep for months.

She urges him to see his doctor at the university health center. He makes the appointment, explains his problem, and is referred to a urologist. The urologist prescribes some medication for him, and while it helps a bit, the side effects are really bothersome. Art goes back to the urologist to discuss an alternative. The urologist explains that this means surgery, "the roto-rooter procedure" that is, a TURP (transurethral resection of the prostate), and Art agrees to have this. The surgery is planned for the winter break, so that he won't miss any teaching.

As men age, the prostate, located underneath the bladder and surrounding the urethra, enlarges and may put pressure on the urethra. This enlargement is called benign (because it is not malignant) prostatic hypertrophy (growth of tissues) or BPH. It leads to the frequent need to pass urine, which is often worse at night, as well as changes to the flow of urine that can be bothersome. While in recent years there have been major advances in the medical treatment of this condition, many men will still have some form of surgery to open up the urethra to correct the pressure and reduce the symptoms. This surgery is commonly called the "roto-rooter" procedure: using surgical tools or lasers, an instrument is inserted into the urethra and advanced to the location where there is excess tissue; the tissue is then removed or burned away. But some men are not able to have the procedure done through the urethra, and then an open prostatectomy needs to be done. In this surgery, an incision is made through the abdomen and the tissue in the prostate itself is removed, but the outer capsule of the prostate remains in the body. This is different from the surgery that is performed to remove the prostate in the case of prostate cancer, which is described in chapter 6.

How Is Sexuality Affected by Surgery to Treat BPH?

Having this surgery increases a man's risk of developing or worsening his erectile functioning. Men may also experience retrograde ejaculation, in which the bladder neck does not close during ejaculation and the fluid flows into the bladder instead of to the outside though the urethra. This may affect the sensation of ejaculation, but most men continue to report sexual satisfaction after the procedure. In men who still want to have children, retrograde ejaculation poses a problem, as the sperm will not pass into the reproductive tract of their partner.

Solutions

Erectile difficulties can be treated with oral medications such as Viagra, Cialis, or Levitra; or men can use more invasive or mechanical erectile aids such as the vacuum pump, the intraurethral pellet, or penile injections to achieve erections sufficient for penetration.

For men who want to have more children, the problems with retrograde ejaculation can be remedied by a fertility specialist, who will be able to take the sperm out of the urine and then perform artificial insemination of the partner or use the sperm to fertilize an egg in the laboratory. The resulting embryo(s) will be transferred to the uterus of the female partner at another time.

Many men find that once their frequent need to urinate decreases, they are more interested in sex and can cope with any erectile problems resulting from the treatment. Getting a decent night's sleep without waking numerous times to go to the bathroom can work wonders for the libido!

CONCLUSION

This chapter has described the sexual issues surrounding surgery of various kinds. Hysterectomy is an extremely common surgery for women, and the sexual side effects cannot be ignored. As the population ages, joint replacement surgery becomes more common. Cardiac surgery is also fairly common in both men and women. As with the medical conditions described in the previous chapter, sexual side effects are not discussed routinely with those having surgery, even though sexual side effects are common.

SUGGESTED READING

Hysterectomy

Haas, A., and S. Puretz. *The Woman's Guide to Hysterectomy.* Berkeley, CA: Celestial Arts, 2002.
Kelley, K. *Through the Land of Hyster: The Hyster Sisters Guide.* Berkeley, CA: Hyster Sisters, 2001.Web Sites

Colon Disease

http://www.ccfa.org/frameviewer/?url=/media/pdf/ibdsexuality.pdf
This is a booklet produced by the Crohn's and Colitis Foundation of America about sexuality and bowel disease.
http://www.uoaa.org/ostomy_info/pubs/uoa_sexuality_en.pdf
This is an online pamphlet produced by the United Ostomy Association in the United States. It contains information about sexuality for the person with a stoma.

Chapter Six

SEXUALITY IN MENTAL ILLNESS

People who struggle with mental illness often have problems with sexual functioning or experience problems as a side effect of the medication prescribed to treat their symptoms. Other people self-medicate with alcohol or other drugs and experience sexual side effects as a result of this. And the intellectually challenged have some special issues related to sexuality. This chapter will highlight the unique sexual effects of mental illness and the medications used to treat them, as well as the effects of recreational drugs on sexual functioning. The special situation of the intellectually challenged will also be addressed.

DEPRESSION AND SEXUALITY

Ruth has struggled with depression most of her life. At 26 years of age she has few friends. She works at the local library and has become very fond of a middle-aged man who is a frequent customer at the library. He is a widow; his wife died three years ago of breast cancer. They talk a lot when he comes to the library, and over time they admit that they have feelings for each other. Ruth is surprised that this has happened to her; she expected that she would remain alone for the rest of her life.

She goes to see a new family physician to get a prescription for birth control pills; she and Gerry have talked about having sex one day and she wants to be prepared. The family doctor asks her how she is feeling overall, and Ruth admits that she is often depressed and that she has lived with depression for most of her life. Dr. Shaw offers her an antidepressant and Ruth thinks that maybe she should try it; maybe it would help.

Depression is a common mental illness that was once shrouded in shame and stigma. In recent years, much of this stigma has disappeared and today, people are much more likely to present to their primary care providers with a request for help with this condition. Women are twice as likely to experience depression than men, and this may start in adolescence. This increased risk may be due to social or biological factors. Women are more frequently affected by physical and sexual abuse; both are risk factors for depression. Poverty is also known to be a precursor to depression, and women are more likely to live in poverty than men. Women are also more likely to experience racial and gender discrimination, which is also implicated in depression. There are also hormonal influences, and it is theorized that the hormonal changes experienced by women across the life span, including the changes associated with pregnancy and menopause, predispose women to cycles of depression.

The experience of depression itself is known to affect sexuality, so much so that at one point the criteria to diagnose depression included both a lack of interest or an increased interest in sex. In fact, almost a third of depressed people who are not treated for their depression report a lack of interest in sex, changes in their usual orgasmic pattern, and difficulty becoming sexually aroused. People with depression may also experience difficulties in their relationships with significant others, which can also contribute to sexual difficulties.

> Ruth has been taking the antidepressant medication for almost three weeks. She notices that her mood is much brighter. In fact, the whole world seems to be much brighter, and she wonders what she has missed all these years. But she has noticed that something else is different; when she and Gerry kiss, she no longer has the same butterfly-in-the-tummy feeling that she used to have. In fact, she hardly even wants to kiss him anymore. This bothers her a lot; she really liked those special times with him.

In the past, depression was usually treated with two kinds of medications: tricyclic antidepressants and monoamine oxidase inhibitors (MAOIs). Both of these were known to cause sexual problems. More recently, newer drugs called selective serotonin reuptake inhibitors (SSRIs) have been shown to be very effective in treating depression. As their use became more popular, those being treated began to report sexual difficulties with these drugs too.

One of the sexual side effects of the SSRIs is a lack of desire for sex. This is complicated to assess, as many people who are depressed report a lack of interest in sex to begin with. If there are other sexual side effects, for example, alterations in an individual's ability to have an orgasm, the lack of interest may be secondary to a lack of satisfaction. But if a person notices a lack of interest in sex that started after he started taking an SSRI, then this is likely a side effect and not something caused by the depression itself. The SSRIs appear to cause an increase in the secretion of the hormone prolactin, which is known to affect libido, especially in men.

Another common side effect of the SSRIs is delayed or absent orgasm. This side effect is so profound that SSRIs are now used to treat rapid ejaculation in men! Some people report that their genitals are less sensitive to touch and stimulation and that this contributes to their lack of arousal. Some men experience erectile dysfunction as a side effect.

The overall incidence of sexual problems in those treated with SSRIs ranges from 50 percent to 90 percent and is a major factor in people stopping their medication early in the treatment; almost 70 percent of those prescribed SSRIs stop taking the medication within the first months of treatment. Different drugs have greater or lesser effects on sexual functioning. Another class of drugs, the serotonin-2 [5-HT2] receptor blockers, appear to cause fewer problems; mirtazapine (Remeron) causes problems in only 24.4 percent and nefazodone (Serzone) in only 8 percent of people on the medication. Men on these medications seem to have more problems than women, but women reported greater severity of problems. All told, 40 percent of those with sexual side effects found this bothersome.

Some other sexual side effects are also seen, including priapism (an erection lasting longer than four hours) in men taking trazadone (Desyrel) and painful orgasm with the tricyclic antidepressants. Some people have reported uncontrollable yawning during orgasm when taking Prozac.

Treatment of Sexual Side Effects

One antidepressant that does not seem to have any sexual side effects is bupropion (Wellbutrin). The addition of this drug to a regimen including any of the other antidepressants appears to lessen the incidence of sexual side effects. This medication may also be used alone to treat depression. Some people even find that when taking bupropion, their sexual interest increases, their level of arousal is also heightened, and they experience more intense orgasms.

Other strategies to deal with the sexual side effects of the antidepressants include waiting for tolerance to the drug to develop (probably the least effective strategy, as most people just stop taking the medication); lowering the dosage of the drug (which may not alleviate the depression); changing to a different type of antidepressant (switching to bupropion may be the best option); or adding an antidote such as sildenafil if the problem is a lack of erections (this is only effective if an antidote exists, which is often not the case). Taking a weekend break from the medication may allow for some alleviation of side effects over the weekend, potentially allowing for improvement for a few days when sexual activity may be attempted.

Some suggest that reassuring the patient that the sexual side effects will disappear once the medication is stopped is another strategy to deal with the side effects, but there are reports of patients in whom the sexual problems persisted for years after stopping the medication. For women with sexual dysfunction from SSRIs, taking the drug sildenafil (Viagra) may improve orgasms.

ANXIETY AND SEXUALITY

John is almost 50 years old and has never had a sexual relationship. His mother always called him her little wallflower and in truth, he never liked to leave the house and had few friends. Today he lives alone in a small apartment not far from his mother. He works at a radio station where he is in charge of the music collection. The job suits him well; he hardly sees anyone and fills the requests that are sent to him by email. He tries to avoid his co-workers, but once or twice a year he has to go to a social event, like the annual Christmas party, and this causes him a great deal of worry. He is afraid that someone will talk to him and he won't know what to say. He is afraid that they will make him play a game and he will make a fool of himself. Last year at the Christmas party he drank too much and was really mortified when he threw up on the steps of the restaurant as he was leaving and he was sure that everyone saw him and laughed.

Social anxiety disorder (SAD) is another common mental illness, with almost 14 percent of adults meeting the criteria for a diagnosis of this disorder at some time in their lives. Slightly more women than men are diagnosed with this disorder. The experience of SAD typically involves a persistent and chronic feeling of being judged by others and/or being embarrassed by one's own actions. Even when the person recognizes that her fears are exaggerated or unreasonable, it is still difficult to overcome them. There are physical symptoms that often go along with the emotional feelings; these include excessive blushing, sweating, trembling, nausea, heart palpitations, and stammering. Some people experience panic attacks that can be both frightening and debilitating. Often people self-medicate with alcohol or recreational drugs in order to function in social situations; this increases their risk of developing a dependency on these substances. Treatment for social anxiety disorder usually includes one of the SSRIs, and so people with anxiety are also susceptible to the same sorts of sexual side effects as those experienced by people with depression.

Buspirone (Buspar) is an antianxiety medication that is sometimes used to treat the sexual side effects associated with the SSRIs. It is used to treat generalized anxiety rather than social anxiety and takes up to three weeks to become effective.

Jeff at the age of 28 has recently started seeing a new woman and he thinks he is in love. His last girlfriend left him about two years ago; she wanted to get married but he was not ready and she told him she wasn't going to waste her time. Nancy is about the same age as Jeff and is the most beautiful woman he has ever seen. In fact, he's not sure why she's interested in him. He can't believe that someone so beautiful and smart and successful would even look at a guy like him.

The first time they went to bed together, Jeff was really nervous. He was nervous all evening and probably drank a bit too much wine with dinner. They were kissing and touching each other in the car outside her apartment, and she invited him in. And nothing happened when they got inside her door. Nothing. Jeff was really upset, but Nancy laughed it off and said it was probably the wine. The next weekend they were at his house watching football and he was careful not to drink at all. But it happened again. Or rather, nothing happened at all. He can understand that it might happen once. But twice?

Anxiety may manifest itself in sexual functioning in both men and women where anxiety develops about the sex act itself, or about components of sexual functioning. For example, some men may become so preoccupied with concerns about their ability to achieve or maintain an erection that they develop performance anxiety, which causes the loss of the erection. This can lead to low self-esteem and avoidance of sexual activity, which in turn causes distancing and loss of intimacy in the relationship. Women can suffer from anxiety related to the way they look when naked or when involved in sexual activity. This preoccupation causes a phenomenon called spectatoring, in which the woman "watches" herself or imagines what she must look like during sexual activity. This can cause tension and an inability to relax, which is a barrier to experiencing sexual pleasure.

Most people with anxiety respond well to cognitive therapy; learning to deal with the triggers that cause anxiety is highly effective. This works for the anxiety associated with sexuality, too. Learning to shut off negative feelings about one's appearance and consciously thinking positive thoughts can help some people who are anxious about what their body looks like. Making an effort to shut off feelings of anxiety about sexual performance works, too. But this is a lifelong endeavor, and some people may prefer a quick fix from medication, even though the medications used for anxiety are the same SSRIs that cause sexual problems of their own.

OBSESSIVE-COMPULSIVE DISORDER

Ronda is a germ freak. She knows it, her family and friends know it. They make jokes about it, about how her home is so clean that you could do surgery on the floor. But it really isn't that funny. It affects her life in really bad ways. She cleans up after her husband all the time, and he seems to be getting more and more irritated with this. She has to clean the bathrooms at home at least three times a day, even the bathroom in the basement that no one uses.

But there's a bigger problem: the thought of sex is really disgusting to her now, and she tries to do whatever she can to get out of it. She starts complaining about being tired as soon as she gets home after work. She tells her husband that she is busy when he goes to bed, and she goes to bed when she knows he's asleep. She even picks a fight after dinner so that he is mad with her at bed time. When she does have sex with him, and she's only done it about three times in the last year, she had to grit her teeth to keep from leaping out of the bed, and afterward, she had to take a really hot shower. The thought of sex makes her feel physically ill, and she can't talk to her husband about it because he just won't understand.

Obsessive-compulsive disorder (OCD) is a chronic anxiety disorder with some unique features: the person commonly has frequent, distressing, intrusive thoughts and may attempt to try to relieve the anxiety by performing repetitive tasks. Some people experience sexually intrusive thoughts: they think obsessively about doing something sexual with another person, and sometimes the sexual act is repulsive to them or the person they think about doing it with is inappropriate, for example, a child. These thoughts can cause a great deal of distress and self-hate.

Studies indicate that women with OCD experience significant challenges in their sexual lives. They are more likely to experience low sexual pleasure, high levels of disgust at the thought of sexual activity or with the act itself, low sexual desire, poor sexual arousal, and a lack of sexual satisfaction. These experiences occur among women with OCD even if they do not have obsessions with cleanliness or contamination, which is a frequent manifestation of the condition (often seen as frequent hand washing or extreme fear of germs). These sexual problems are seen independent of the side effects of medication and may be an integral part of the condition for some women.

This is a condition that is often treated with the SSRI family of drugs, and so the person may experience any and all of the side effects associated with these medications. There is some controversy about the effectiveness of these drugs for this condition. Some people find relief in cognitive-behavioral therapy, where they learn to control the obsessive thoughts and feelings that cause so much distress and interfere with family and social functioning.

SCHIZOPHRENIA

Schizophrenia is a condition in which the perception of reality is altered. A person with this condition may experience auditory hallucinations, delusional thinking that is often paranoid, or thoughts that are confused. The person usually experiences a significant breakdown in family, social, and occupational relationships. Schizophrenia has a profound effect on the ability of affected individuals to interact in society and they are often marginalized. The onset of this condition is usually in the middle to late twenties, and men and women are equally affected. Because of the challenges in maintaining relationships, schizophrenics often do not have meaningful long-term relationships with a significant other. This can affect their access to regular sexual activity. In addition, many have sexual difficulties as a result of the illness itself: one of the manifestations of the disease is a lack of ability to enjoy pleasure, and so individuals are not able to enjoy sex, if and when they are able to have it.

Treatment usually involves neuroleptic medications (phenothiazines, butyrophenones, and thioxanthines) that have significant sexual side effects. These side effects are usually dose related. In men, erectile difficulties are common; however, some men may experience priapism when on these drugs. Priapism is considered a medical emergency and men should seek medical attention to prevent permanent damage to the tissues of the penis. This can present challenges to the man who is suffering from these symptoms and may not recognize that something is wrong, may not remember to go to the hospital, or may be afraid to seek help. In women on neuroleptics, arousal difficulties include poor vaginal lubrication and diminished or absent orgasms.

Another class of medications may be used to treat schizophrenic patients: atypical antipsychotics such as olanzapine (Zyprex), risperidone (Risperdal), and clozaine (Clozaril). All of these have sexual side effects, including delayed or absent ejaculation in men and breast tenderness in women.

SUBSTANCE ABUSE AND SEXUALITY

Sandy has had a rough life. She was thrown out of her home at the age of 15, when her mother took up with a new boyfriend who tried to touch Sandy's breasts. When Sandy complained, her mother accused her of trying to ruin her mother's life. Sandy lived with a friend for a while but then moved in with her own boyfriend. They had always used marijuana, but over time, her boyfriend started using cocaine, and when that got too expensive, he switched to oxycontin and then to heroin. He tried to persuade Sandy to use with him but she was too scared, and besides, she was the one who had a job and brought in the money that paid for his drugs.

When he was high, he frequently demanded sex from her. Even when she was tired and even when she was asleep, he would badger her and eventually she would just give in to try and get it over with. But it was not easy. He would lose his erection quickly and demand oral sex so that he could get hard again. This could go on for a long time, and if she complained or tried to stop, he would threaten her. Once he even grabbed her hair and pulled her head to his lap. That scared her, but she thought it was not his fault, that he was high and didn't know what he was doing.

It is well known that the use of alcohol and recreational drugs affects sexuality for both men and women. Many people assume that intoxicants such as alcohol and drugs improve sexual functioning, but this is a perception that is not borne out in reality. While being high or drunk may make people feel as if they are aroused, in reality their sexual performance is diminished. With chronic use, drugs and alcohol decrease physical arousal, reduce the capacity for orgasm, and decrease libido. The effect of the drugs is dependent on the type of drug used, the amount used, and the length of time for which the drug is taken.

Alcohol tends to lessen inhibitions and has also been used for many centuries as an aphrodisiac. While many people believe that alcohol intensifies the sexual response, it in fact impairs response; but under the influence, many people are less inhibited and thus more likely to engage in sexual activity or to be less inhibited during such activity. The acute effects of alcohol can interfere with erections and vaginal lubrication as well as orgasm for both men and women. Abuse of alcohol often causes relationship problems, and sexual problems may result from this.

Marijuana has historically been used as a sexual enhancer in many different cultures. It is perceived as improving sexual functioning by increasing sexual pleasure and enhancing libido. As with many other recreational drugs, when increasing amounts of the drug are used the positive effects tend to decrease.

Cocaine increases feelings of well-being and may enhance libido in the short term. It is known to cause improved erections, faster ejaculation, and more intense orgasms initially, but with long-term use it may cause difficulty in achieving an erection and ejaculating. Some men may not recover sexual function even after the drug use is halted. Women who use cocaine also have problems achieving orgasm after long-term use and experience low sexual desire.

Opiates such as heroin and morphine have a negative effect on arousal for both men and women. These drugs direct blood away from the genitals and thus make orgasm difficult to achieve. In men, opiate use decreases testosterone levels and contributes to low sexual desire. But some men like the effect that these drugs have on the length of time they last before orgasm and so use it to delay orgasm. These drugs tend to cause relaxation, so for some women the use of opiates may relax them and reduce pain during penetration. The acute rush from taking heroin produces sensations of intense pleasure, sometimes described as a pharmacologic orgasm. This sensation can in itself be addicting.

When people try to withdraw from taking opiates, they can also experience sexual problems. Hypersexuality is common in men who are withdrawing from these drugs, and they may experience premature ejaculation and multiple erections throughout the day and night.

Amphetamines have the reputation of improving all aspects of the sexual response, including increasing libido, intensifying orgasm, and making the sexual encounter last longer. This may be true when they are taken in low doses, but these drugs are very addicting and soon users increase both the dose that they use as well as the frequency of use. This has a negative impact on sexual functioning, with users experiencing an inability to achieve orgasm and a lack of interest in sex.

Methamphetamine, a popular form of amphetamine, is used as a party drug and is known to increase social confidence, increase energy, and cause sexual disinhibition. These effects all increase sexual activity and hence explain the drug's popularity at parties. Because sex while under the influence of this drug is so pleasurable, the use of the drug becomes strongly associated with sex and thus becomes psychologically addicting in addition to the physiological addiction. People who are high or drunk do not use condoms consistently, thus putting themselves at risk for sexually transmitted infections (STIs) and HIV. Women may be more likely to have unprotected sex and be at risk of pregnancy in addition to STIs. Being high may improve people's perception of themselves as attractive and outgoing, and they may actually act that way, but being high also increases the chances of engaging in risky sexual behavior, which in turn poses a very real threat to health.

Chronic use of amphetamines results in ED and delayed orgasm in men and delayed or absent orgasm in women. There is also a condition in men termed "crystal dick," in which men on methamphetamines have high libido, high energy, and disinhibition but are unable to have an erection.

Ecstasy is another party drug that has a stimulant effect; it is known as the "love drug." People who take this drug describe feelings of increased sexual desire and also report increased sexual satisfaction from sexual activity when they are high. Orgasm is usually delayed for both men and women, and some men have difficulty achieving an erection when on this drug. There have also been reports of men experiencing priapism while on Ecstasy.

Ecstasy is sometimes taken with sildenafil; this combination is called "sextasy" and is reported also to increase desire and enhance sexual pleasure. Sildenafil causes a drop in blood pressure and can be dangerous for some people; it can also be dangerous when used in combination with street drugs.

Poppers are drugs that cause dilation of blood vessels. The drugs come in an ampoule or small bottle and when this is opened, vapors containing nitrous oxide are released. When this is inhaled, it causes a rush in which a sense of euphoria and relaxation is felt. These drugs are often used to facilitate anal intercourse where relaxation of the anal sphincter is needed to allow penetration. When sildenafil is taken at the same time as poppers, the combination of the two drugs may cause a dangerous drop in blood pressure, heart attack, or stroke.

Drugs Used to Enhance Sex

Some people may use drugs to overcome sexual difficulties. In a study of men who had previously used a variety of drugs including heroin, cocaine, and marijuana, 44 percent had used them to try to lessen sexual difficulties. These included erectile dysfunction, premature ejaculation, and low sexual desire. The men in this study ranged in age from 22 to 35 years, which is quite young to have these kinds of sexual problems. These men were self-medicating in an attempt to overcome the embarrassment of having some sort of sexual problem and improve their sexual performance.

Women are also susceptible to these kinds of beliefs. In a study of women who had previously used drugs such as heroin and cocaine, it was found that some believed that the drugs enhanced their sexual performance, increased their libido, and enhanced their pleasure. But among those who used cocaine, there was a recognition that the drugs actually inhibited their desire and sexual performance. When asked about the influence of drugs on their male sexual partners, the women said they believed that heroin and cocaine improved their performance but also that the drugs increased abusive and coercive behavior that ultimately affected the relationship.

INTELLECTUAL DISABILITY

> Sharon is 33 years old and has Down syndrome. She lives at home with her mother and is able to dress herself with help but requires assistance with all her hygiene activities. She likes to sleep in her mother's bed; she has always done this, and for many years her mother has allowed it. But her mother is now in her late sixties and has been advised to start thinking about a residential placement for Sharon.
> It has been difficult for Sharon's mother to force her daughter to sleep in her own bed. Sharon cries and comes to her mother's room repeatedly during the night. And for the last month or more, her mother has noticed that Sharon is touching herself "down there" when she is in her own bed. This bothers her mother, and she asks the social worker what she can do to stop this behavior.

Men and women who are intellectually disabled experience the same sexual needs and desires as the general population. But the way those needs are met is very different. For many years, the focus of any attention to the sexual lives of the intellectually disabled was on the prevention of pregnancy in girls and women, and the threat of sexual abuse of both men and women. It is now recognized that the intellectually disabled have the right to sexual pleasure; the greatest challenge to this is the attitudes of others, in particular parents, who may be fearful that their children will be harmed by it. People with intellectual disabilities have traditionally been viewed as being asexual, childlike, oversexed, or likely to become sexual offenders. It has been suggested that proof of inappropriate sexual activity lies in instances where an intellectually disabled man or woman masturbates, perhaps excessively in the eyes of care providers. But masturbation is often the only form of sexual expression available to those with intellectual disabilities; however, it is viewed as pathological instead of as a normal and natural experience as it is for the general population. Masturbation is problematic when it occurs in public, when it occurs for prolonged periods of time, and when it causes injury to the person masturbating, due to excessive force or prolonged stimulation.

People with intellectual disabilities can be taught that there is a time and place for masturbation, in much the same way that they are taught not to burp or pass gas in public. These lessons may have to be taught over and over, and it is often a reflection of parents' or caregivers' discomfort with the topic and activity rather than the capacity of the person with an intellectual disability that this is seen as too much of a challenge.

People with intellectual disabilities have historically been the victims of unwanted sexual touching and even sexual abuse. This may occur at the hands of family members, caregivers, or other people living in the same institutions. Sexual abuse may lead to self-injury or inappropriate sexual touching of self or others as a response to the abuse, especially for people who are nonverbal and cannot relate what has happened to them.

CONCLUSION

This chapter has described the sexual issues related to depression and anxiety, and to other mental illnesses such as obsessive compulsive disorder and schizophrenia. The effects of abuse of alcohol and other recreational or street drugs has also been discussed. Finally, the challenges for the intellectually disabled have been presented.

WEB SITES

http://www.cmha.ca/bins/content_page.asp?cid=3&lang=1
This is the official Web site of the Canadian Mental Health Association. It has resources for people with mental illness as well as for their family and friends. There are also links to some resources on sexuality and mental illness.
http://cartercenter.org/health/mental_health/index.html?gclid=CJHMveLrl5YCFRLoxg odWUFZnA
This is the Web site of the Carter Center, started by President Jimmy Carter and his wife. The center has a strong mental health program, which aims to reduce the stigma associated with mental illness around the world.

Chapter Seven

SEXUALITY FOLLOWING COMBAT INJURY

Traumatic injury often affects young people who have not yet established primary intimate relationships or are exploring new aspects of their sexual selves. But when a traumatic injury occurs, regardless of the age of the person or the type of trauma, the immediate concerns are for the person's survival. It's in the weeks, months, and years after recovery from the injury that other lifestyle considerations come into play, and these of course include sexuality and sexual functioning. This is of special importance in the armed forces, where tens of thousands of young men and women are injured in combat in war zones.

COMBAT INJURIES

When someone is injured in combat, the resultant alterations in sexuality are variable. There may be changes in some or all aspects of the normal sexual response cycle including desire, arousal, orgasm, and satisfaction. Brain injury may result in changes in sexual thoughts and feelings. When limbs have been lost or severely damaged, there may be changes in the mechanics of sex. An injured veteran may have difficulty establishing new sexual relationships with an altered body. And also of importance is the effect of all this on the sexual partner in response to any and all of these changes. And these are mostly physical effects. The changes as a result of posttraumatic stress disorder (PTSD) have far-reaching consequences for the combat veteran and his or her partner. These changes influence emotions and adjustment in all aspects of social and sexual life.

Traumatic Brain Injury and Posttraumatic Stress Disorder

Jason went to fight in Iraq with the determination and confidence of a warrior. He'd been trained in reconnaissance and was eager to get into the field of battle and do his job. Three months before being deployed, Jason met Michelle and they fell in love almost instantly. With the date of his departure coming ever closer, Jason proposed one sunny day when they were walking near his parents' cottage at the lake. Michelle was surprised but happy and agreed that they would be married when he returned from his tour of duty.

Six weeks later, Jason was injured when an explosive device detonated under the armed vehicle in which he was riding on a lonely road on the outskirts of Baghdad. No one in the vehicle saw it coming, and minutes after the blast the air was filled with smoke and screams and the metallic smell of burned flesh and blood. Everyone in the vehicle was injured, but Jason was the worst. He was evacuated from the scene and flown by helicopter to the base. Within hours he was on his way to the medical center in Germany, and that's where he woke up for the first time.

He wasn't sure what had happened; his last memory was of the hot sun shining in through the windows of the armored vehicle. It took him some time after he woke up to figure out what had happened and where he was. Mostly what he felt was pain, a searing, burning pain all over his body that was there even though he knew the nurses were giving him pain medication. His head felt woozy—almost as if he was drunk or high—and the nausea came in waves.

Two days and three surgeries later he was shipped back to the United States. He vaguely remembered being told that he had burns all over his body and his leg was shattered. At least, that's what he thought he heard. He was still in a fog and the pain was so bad. He thought about seeing Michelle again. But then a dark thought crept into his brain: what if she didn't want him anymore? This time the pain was inside, deep in the center of him, and he thought about it all the time.

Michelle arrived at the hospital within 24 hours of his arrival there. At first he wouldn't talk to her, and he lay with his eyes closed, his head turned away. Most of his face was bandaged and she could only see his eyes, dark and angry. Every now and then Jason had outbursts of terrible anger; Michelle didn't know how to react, as the man she knew was kind and gentle. During these outbursts, he threw himself around the bed, tried to rip out his IV lines, and hit his hands repeatedly on the bed rails. When this happened, the nurses rushed over and gave him heavy doses of sedation. He eventually passed out for a couple of hours after that, and then it began again: the blaming and the harsh words and the swearing and eventually the anger and violence.

Traumatic brain injury (TBI) may affect sexual functioning in a variety of ways. In the acute stage, when injured service members are in hospital, it is not uncommon for them to display sexual behaviors that are unusual for them. They may resist wearing clothing and may tear off their bedclothes and attempt to move around naked. This is disconcerting to the family, although staff members are usually quite used to this and will deal with it in a matter-of-fact way.

The location of the injury has an influence on the sexual side effects experienced. Disinhibition (lack of the usual filters that control behavior) is a common side effect of brain injury, particularly injury to the frontal lobe. The injured person may masturbate in full view of staff or other patients and may do this repeatedly. The person may also be hypersexual and may make sexual advances to a partner and/or staff members. These behaviors are called sexually intrusive behaviors and cause a great deal of distress to family members. They are usually worse soon after the injury and do improve over time. Damage to the temporal lobe may cause a lack of interest in sex and alterations in genital arousal. Damage to the pituitary gland may result in alterations in hormone production and in men may cause a decrease in androgen levels, resulting in erectile difficulty and a lack of interest in sex.

Brain injuries often result in extreme mood fluctuations, anxiety, and depression. Some people with brain injuries lose the capacity to interpret social cues and so may act inappropriately in social situations, causing embarrassment to themselves and to their partners and family members.

Brain injuries may lead to personality changes, and partners may find that the person they fell in love with is not the person who has come back from war. This can cause significant problems for partners, who may not be "in love" with this changed person, who looks like their partner but acts differently. If brain-injured persons make excessive sexual demands of their partners, this can be especially difficult. The sexual demands are often not accompanied by the usual emotional outreach, and so there is discordance for partners, which can be very distressing. If the brain injury results in a lack of interest in sex, partners may be left feeling isolated and without affection. If a partner is providing a great deal of physical support, this can be an additional loss. The partner provides intimate physical care but receives little in response.

Some men with TBI report difficulties with erections. The cause of this is not clear. It may be because of loss of sensation due to brain damage or perhaps because of difficulty communicating with the partner, leading to withdrawal. A more likely cause, however, is the brain-injured person's mood, with irritability and altered concentration contributing to distraction, which alters the response to sexual touch. Feeling unattractive due to scars can also make the injured person feel less sexually attractive, which may cause erectile difficulties. There are reports of female veterans having difficulties with sexual response; however, most reports are of male combat veterans.

Closed head injuries may occur when a service member experiences an explosion with minimal or no external injury because he is wearing a helmet. Even though nothing appears to be wrong, the force of the brain moving in the skull can cause significant damage and side effects. Up to 50 percent of men who have this kind of injury will experience symptoms that can impair sexual functioning. These include irritability, depression, and anxiety. People with closed head injuries may also have difficulty expressing themselves, particularly in the emotional area, and relationships may suffer as a result. Closed head injuries are invisible injuries, and many report that they receive little attention as they do not appear to be injured.

Many of the medications used to treat TBI cause sexual problems. Antidepressants, antipsychotics, anticonvulsants, and anticholinergic drugs may all affect libido, and many also affect orgasm and ejaculation.

> Jason remained in the military hospital for two months while his body healed. His leg healed fastest, although he still couldn't walk unassisted. They'd told him that his thigh bone was shattered and that there was a really bad infection deep in the wound. The burns took longer to heal; he had to wear tight constriction garments all over, including his face, and he had yet to look at himself in the mirror.
>
> But the nights were the worst. In the darkness of his room, the dreams came. Any noise could set them off. A door banging, a whisper outside his room, and he was instantly back in Iraq, with its dusty streets and dangers. His dreams were full of the sounds and smells of war and terror and blood and death.
>
> One morning, Michelle came into his room while he was sleeping and touched him on his shoulder. He grabbed hold of her arm and twisted it behind her back so fast she didn't even have time to scream. It was as if he was possessed and she struggled to release herself. "Bitch," he shouted, "F—ing bitch! Suck my —, bitch. Go on, do it!" By now the nurses were in the room, and one of them led Michelle away.

PTSD may also play an important role in changes in sexual thoughts and feelings. Many veterans have seen violent attacks on civilians as part of their tour of duty. They may also have witnessed sexual assaults and torture. As one veteran stated, "Night goggles allow us to see things that should not be seen. On patrol at night I have seen women and men being assaulted. The sights are now part of my nightmares." Sexual activity may act as a trigger for flashbacks when the sounds and smells associated with sex remind the veteran of things witnessed while on duty. Men with PTSD have also been shown to be more aggressive toward their intimate partners; this aggression may be physical, verbal, or psychological. Aggression can then spill over into the sexual relationship, which is distressing.

PTSD is known to cause problems with multiple aspects of sexual functioning. It is associated with erectile difficulties in many men; up to 85 percent of men with PTSD may have ongoing problems achieving and maintaining an erection. Treatment with sildenafil (Viagra) has been shown to improve this. PTSD is also associated with lowered sexual desire and problems with orgasm and overall sexual satisfaction. Many of those suffering from PTSD are prescribed antidepressants, specifically the selective serotonin reuptake inhibitors (SSRIs). While these are effective in treating many of the symptoms of PTSD, they are also known to cause sexual dysfunction, particularly in libido, arousal, and orgasm, thus making the sexual side effects of the condition even worse.

Injured veterans may have suffered significant physical changes, and these may affect body image, which in turn affects self-esteem and sexual self-image. People with severe physical injuries may not see themselves as sexually attractive. Amputees are known to experience anxiety, depression, and discomfort in social situations and anxiety about body image. All of these may impact on a healthy sexual self-concept and normal sexual functioning.

Changes in the Mechanics of Sex

Jason spent a long time in the rehab hospital. He was taking medication to help with his PTSD and it seemed to be working. He was much less angry, and the bad dreams seemed to have gone away. It helped if he slept with the light on. Eventually he was able to walk with a cane and he went home. He still had to wear constriction garments on his head, face, and torso; they told him this was to limit the scarring from the burns. He hated them; they were hot and tight and took a lot of effort to remove for his daily shower and then put on again. He needed help with this and now that he was home, Michelle had to do it. He hated her to see him like this. He wondered what she really thought of him now. He needed help with so many things, and he couldn't even kiss her properly with the constriction bandages on his face. He wondered why she was even sticking around.

Due to improved surgical techniques and speedier evacuation of wounded personnel, soldiers today are being saved when previously they had succumbed to their injuries. But they are surviving with injuries that are at times very significant. Soldiers are surviving with the loss of two or more limbs. Some suffer significant burns over large areas of their bodies. The types of injuries seen in today's combat veterans are the result of improvised explosive devices (IEDs), mortars, and rocket-propelled grenades. These all produce fragment wounds that can't be prevented, even with body armor.

Depending on the physical damage from combat injuries, challenges to the mechanical aspects of sexual activity may result. These refer specifically to sexual positioning and sexual technique. Bony injuries or amputations can alter a person's ability to balance during sexual activity. Contractures after burns can limit mobility, especially joint mobility. Nerve damage after any kind of injury can also affect posture and balance, and nerve pain with or without pressure on affected parts can be limiting as well.

Amputation of one or more limbs can have a profound affect on the mechanics of sex as well as on body image. Many people with amputations have never talked to anyone about the effect on their sex life. Very little research has been done on this topic, but one study showed that men with amputations have significant sexual issues and have problems achieving erections and also with orgasms. The reasons for this were not explained in the study. A man with one or both above knee amputations may have problems at times maintaining balance during sexual intercourse if he is on top. Thrusting during intercourse may place pressure on the stump(s) and may cause pain that can interfere with sexual pleasure. If the partner is on top, these issues may be prevented, but this may limit the types of positions that can be used and may cause dissatisfaction for some couples. Similarly, if the veteran is a woman with a lower leg amputation, she may not be able to be on top during sex, as she may not have sufficient balance to maintain this position. Loss of an upper limb may also affect balance, but it will certainly affect touching during sex. Learning to use another hand to stimulate yourself or your partner can be very challenging. Most of us use our dominant hand to touch our own bodies or those of our partners, and using the other hand can feel awkward. But this can be a good thing, as novelty may heighten sensation.

Anything we know about changes in sexual function in a person with *burns* has been learned from the general population and not from those injured in combat. But we do know that after a significant burn with resulting scarring, there are concerns about body image and self-esteem. Many burn victims also suffer from PTSD and have difficulty adjusting to life after the incident. Many people with severe burns are treated with antidepressants and antianxiety medications, all of which have sexual side effects. The permanent skin contractures and nerve damage from the burn may also result in chronic pain. This can greatly influence the mechanics of sex. Think about a man who has extensive burns to his lower body with scar tissue and contractures on his hips and upper thighs. He may not be able to bend his hips easily, and so intercourse in the missionary position will be difficult for him and perhaps even painful. There may even be problems if he is on the bottom and his partner on top, as the contractures may prevent him from being able to lie flat on the bed. Men or women with upper body burns may have scars and contractures preventing them from being able to hold their partner in their arms. Burns to the face may prevent kissing, and the scar tissue usually has little sensation so people with the burns may not be able to feel the caress or kiss of their partners.

Trauma to the genital area presents a unique set of physical and psychological challenges to combat veterans and their partners. Damage to tissue in this area may result in loss of function or anatomical changes that make normal sexual activity very difficult. For a man, trauma to the genital area may mean the partial or total loss of the penis and/or testicles. This has obvious serious consequences for fertility and sexuality. But even if the penis and/or testicles have not been destroyed, scarring and nerve damage may affect the functioning of those organs. For a woman who has been injured, the injuries themselves or the side effects of surgery and other treatments may also alter the anatomy and functioning of the sexual organs including the vulva, clitoris, and vagina. Nerve damage may alter sensations even if the anatomy has been restored, and what was previously perceived as a pleasurable sensation may now be felt as painful. The loss of reproductive potential if the testicles or uterus have been damaged may also have consequences in the sexual realm; some people may be reluctant to be sexually active if they are unable to conceive. These are not rational decisions, but they reflect the enormity of the psychological and emotional damage from a devastating injury.

Body image issues are also significant, and injured individuals and their partners may need extensive sex therapy to overcome the many challenges they will face. Body image issues include the perception of the altered self as well as some real challenges to being sexual when the genitals have been severely damaged or destroyed.

> Things didn't improve between Jason and Michelle. She tried to tell him that she loved him, and he told her he didn't believe her. She tried to show him that she loved him in so many different ways and he just pushed her away. And one day she went. Jason was sad for a while and then his sadness turned to anger. He didn't need her or anyone else for that matter!
>
> After a couple of weeks Jason was really lonely. Outside of his daily rehab visits, he was all alone. His friends from his unit were still in Iraq, and his friends from high school were busy with their lives. They were all married and some of them had new babies. The only women he met were nurses and physiotherapists and doctors. And none of them even looked at him as a man, just as a bashed up soldier.

Changes in Access to Sexual Activity

Returning veterans who have been injured or who experience a relationship breakdown after returning from combat face additional challenges in connecting with new partners. Challenges to body image often affect self-confidence, and the injured veterans may think of themselves as unattractive and unable to find someone to love them. Long periods of rehabilitation may mean that they have limited opportunities to meet new partners. We know from the amputee community that younger people with amputations have less social contact with friends and relatives than their unaffected peers and are less likely to go to movies, sporting events, and dances, all of which are situations where they can meet others. These restrictions may be self-imposed, as veterans refuse social contact due to reluctance to connect with those who knew them before the combat injury. For those with PTSD it is even more difficult to engage socially, and these veterans are even more likely to withdraw from social contact.

Relationship Changes

The partner of the injured soldier is intimately involved in all the changes experienced. There is potential for significant distress in both the sexual and the emotional relationship; this has been seen among veterans and their partners since the Vietnam War. When a partner returns home injured, the priority may not be the sexual relationship. Coping with the immediate challenges is usually the most important activity for the partner, while at the same time keeping things normal for any children. However, sexuality does tend to come to the forefront at some point in the recovery process. Sexual activity may be seen by one of those involved as a luxury rather than a priority, while for the other it may be a critical component of a return to normality. This applies to either the injured veteran or the partner. It is difficult to anticipate who may be reluctant and for what reasons.

Challenges to sexuality are particularly important for the couple in cases where brain injury has occurred. Traumatic brain injury can disrupt existing relationships, because personality changes fundamentally affect how the couple functions in all areas of life together. Difficulties with communication may complicate any sexual problems experienced by the couple. This is particularly pertinent to veterans who have sustained a brain injury, as their reasoning capacity may be affected, or they may be experiencing sexual impulsivity and may not understand why their partner refuses their demands for sex. If the couple was not able to talk about sex easily before the injury, it may be very difficult to talk about it when there are real physical and emotional issues to deal with.

Caring for someone who has sustained multiple physical injuries also poses challenges to a sexual relationship. Making the transition from care provider to sexual partner is particularly challenging when the partner has been assisting with personal hygiene activities. Other challenges relate to the changes experienced by the partner when the service member was deployed. The partner may have made new friendships and found new ways of coping as a single person instead of as part of a couple. The responsibility of sole parenting during the absence of the partner may also affect the relationship when the service member returns. This may cause emotional distance, which can impact on sexual closeness and communication.

Solutions

Solutions to these problems depend on the reason why the problem is occurring. If pain is an issue, the veteran needs to find pain medication that gives relief with minimal side effects. This can be a challenge for sexual activity, as pain medication is often sedating and those who are taking the medication find themselves falling asleep during sex! Taking the medication just before sexual activity can help with this.

For the person with an amputation or scarring that limits the usual sexual positions, the obvious answer is to change the positions used in intercourse. This may be more difficult than it seems, especially if balance and coordination are also affected by the loss of limbs. Many couples have patterns of sexual behavior that have become quite ingrained over the years and may find that making changes is challenging. Negotiating what changes can be made also requires open communication about sexual issues; all this can also be quite challenging and is influenced by age, ethnicity, religious beliefs, and so forth.

When nerve damage has occurred as a result of an injury, actions that were pleasurable before may now be painful; also the injured individual may be dealing with chronic pain at the site of the injury. The injured individual and the partner may need to find new ways to stimulate each other that avoid touching or putting pressure on the part of the body that is painful. This may present a challenge if the injury, for example, is to the hands or the genital area.

In the case of amputation, it is easy to see that new ways of being sexual need to found. A right-handed man whose right arm has been amputated may have to learn new ways to stimulate both himself and his partner. This forces the individual and the couple to be more creative; at times, this may seem overwhelming given all the other changes that have occurred. Sex, once a source of pleasure and comfort, is now another area where changes must be made. Spontaneity must give way to planning and adaptation.

Many injured veterans find it difficult to access services that will help them with sexual problems. It may be daunting to bring up the subject, particularly in an environment where coping and strength are valued. Admitting to a problem is difficult, especially if the veteran is the one who has to bring up the topic.

For the single soldier, the challenges are even greater. Personality changes and difficulties with communication can may make social occasions and dating very difficult. The veteran may need to learn new social skills in order to function in social situations including dating or sexual relationships.

A referral to a sex therapist or counselor can be very helpful for individuals or couples who are having difficulties with the physical and emotional aspects of sex after injury. But it is becoming recognized that this is a significant problem, and in 2008 a one-day meeting was held in Washington, DC, to address the issues of sexuality in this population. It is anticipated that this meeting will begin a process in which sexual problems among injured veterans will be recognized and treated.

CONCLUSION

Combat injuries have the potential to cause significant physical and psychological damage, which will effect sexual functioning as well as the relationship the service member has with the partner. This is something that has been largely ignored, but there are initiatives underway to recognize the sexual consequences of combat injury and to provide support to injured veterans and their partners.

WEB SITES

http://www.saluteheroes.org/
Salute America's Heroes is an organization that provides financial and other support to injured veterans and their families. Every year it organizes a special meeting, called "Road to Recovery," that veterans can apply to attend.
http://www.kaisernetwork.org/health_cast/hcast_index.cfm?display=detail&hc=2570
The Morehouse School of Medicine sponsored a one-day meeting to address the issue of sexuality and injured veterans. The Web site houses audio and video feeds of the day's proceedings.

Chapter Eight

SEXUALITY FOLLOWING SPINAL CORD INJURY

Hundreds of thousands of people are injured in accidents each year. Spinal cord injury devastates the lives of those affected, including their sexual lives. This chapter describes how sexuality is affected by spinal cord and other traumatic injuries.

SPINAL CORD INJURY

Spinal cord injury affects about 250,000 people in the United States, with more than 10,000 new cases occurring each year. Most of these injuries are caused by direct trauma to the spinal cord, and young men under the age of 25 are most likely to suffer this type of injury. In addition to the paralysis that occurs as a result of the damage to the spinal cord, people with this type of injury also have problems controlling bladder and bowel function, and their sexual functioning is also affected. The severity of the problems experienced are in part dictated by the level of the injury and whether the spinal cord is completely severed or not.

Effects on Men

Brian was an athlete in the old days. There wasn't a game he wouldn't play, a mountain he wouldn't climb, or a river he wouldn't cross. And he loved to dive off cliffs into rivers or lakes or oceans. And one day he flew off one such cliff and broke his neck. In an instant his life was changed.

The first couple of weeks in the hospital he was pretty much in shock. He remembered little about his accident other than the feel of the air as he launched himself off the cliff. And now every waking moment was filled with anger and despair. He went from one emotion to the other, cycling between the two frequently and without warning. The anger was better than the despair. The anger at least gave him energy. The despair just felt like a black hole.

He had so many questions: When could he go back to college? Could he still live in his apartment? What about sex? He'd heard some of the other guys on the ward joking about it, but he wasn't sure if they were just fooling around or if they meant what they said.

Most men with a spinal cord injury have difficulty achieving and maintaining an erection. There are two kinds of erections: those resulting from sexual thoughts and images (these are called psychogenic erections) and those that are caused by physical stimulation of the penis (reflex erections). These two mechanisms usually work together to produce and maintain an erection.

Psychogenic erections are controlled higher up in the spinal cord at the T10 to L2 level. Men can have erections by thinking about sex and have to maintain mental sexual arousal in order to physically maintain an erection. Reflex erections are mediated in the spinal cord by a reflex arc in the sacral area (S2 to S4). Spinal cord injury above the sacral level preserves reflex erections and may even allow them to last longer than before. Many men with high-level spinal cord lesions are able to have erections when the penis is touched by clothing or when the bladder is catheterized.

Recovery of sexual function may occur within the first year after the injury in about 70 percent of men, but erectile capacity may never be normal. Those with higher-level lesions recover faster than those with lesions lower in the spinal cord. Spinal cord injury also affects ejaculation, and even in men who are able to achieve an assisted erection, ejaculation is not likely to occur. This may affect sexual pleasure and satisfaction and certainly has a significant impact on fertility. The experience of orgasm in men with spinal cord injury is variable; once again, this is dependent on the level of the injury and whether the spinal cord was completely severed. Even men who do not experience ejaculation may be able to experience the pleasurable sensations of orgasm. In contrast, men who are able to have reflex erections may not be able to experience the pleasurable sensations of orgasm.

A spinal cord injury is devastating to anyone but particularly for young men who are at their peak of sexual functioning. The immediate postinjury period may be fraught with anger and frustration. All this impact on sexual functioning. Depression is common in the early days and weeks following a traumatic injury, and may be compounded by the realization of what has been lost.

Spinal cord injury also affects bladder and bowel control, and leakage of both urine and feces is possible during sexual activity. Men seem to be less bothered by this than women, as we shall discuss later, but the time needed to empty both bladder and bowel before sexual activity as well as the fear of incontinence may also affect sexual desire.

A man with upper and lower limb paralysis may also be unable to support himself on his arms, and this limits the options for positioning for sexual activity. Also, he may not be able to move his hips for thrusting. Some people also experience muscle spasms that interfere with sexual activity and pleasure.

Effects on Women

Paula was riding on the back of her boyfriend's Harley motorcycle when they skidded on some gravel and went down. He was thrown clear and got away with only some scrapes and a broken collarbone. Paula was not that lucky. Her shoe got stuck behind the tailpipe, and the bike fell right on top of her. She had bad burns to her foot, and her spine was broken. After many months of rehab she was able to go home in a wheelchair. While she was in hospital, her boyfriend Gary had renovated their house. He widened all the doorways and lowered the counters in the kitchen. He even turned the den into a new bedroom for them so that everything was on one floor. He'd installed a new shower in the downstairs bathroom, and she could just wheel herself into the shower and transfer to the bench.

Six months after the accident, Paula was adapting very well. She had always been fit, and all those hours in the gym seemed to be paying off; she was able to use her wheelchair with ease and transferring herself from chair to bed was relatively easy.

Gary had been pestering her for sex ever since she got out of the hospital. She'd put him off in the beginning, but after all these months, her excuses seemed to be pretty weak. But she really didn't feel like sex any more and even thought that Gary was pretty strange, still wanting her after everything that had happened. She was worried about her bladder and having an accident; she still had some leakage every now and then, and this really bothered her. But he was insistent and he'd been so good to her since the accident. Maybe she should just let him. . . .

Our knowledge about women with spinal cord injury is somewhat limited by the fact that three times as many men suffer this injury than do women. A lot of the research into women and spinal cord injury has focused on fertility issues rather than sexual issues, but there are some changes that have been described.

Many women with a spinal cord injury, especially those who are partnered at the time of the trauma, report that they have sexual intercourse although not with the frequency that they did before. They also describe problems with finding a comfortable position for both foreplay and intercourse as well as problems with muscle spasms that interfere with the activity. But women are also able to have intercourse even if they are not interested or not aroused. A woman can be the passive recipient of intercourse, and this may account for the frequency of intercourse reported in women with spinal cord injury while levels of satisfaction are not as high. Women who have genital sensation are more satisfied with their sex life than those who don't.

As with men, the level of the injury dictates the impact on sexual functioning. Damage above the S2 to S4 level will allow for vaginal lubrication with stimulation. Damage above the S2 to S4 level of the spinal cord will, however, impact negatively on orgasm. If the woman has genital sensation she is more likely to be able to have an orgasm, but it may require more direct stimulation of greater intensity than before.

Women with spinal cord injury report a lack of desire for sex that is associated with negative body image, depression, low self-esteem, mobility issues, and pain, among other issues related to altered sexual functioning. However, women with spinal cord injury report that they enjoy kissing, hugging, and touching of the entire body, including areas with no sensation.

Women, by virtue of the anatomical placement of the vagina between the urethra and anus, are likely to experience the involuntary loss of urine and/or feces during intercourse. This is extremely bothersome, and some women are reluctant to have intercourse out of fear that this will happen. Emptying both the bladder and bowel before sexual activity may reduce the risk of this happening, but it is not a guarantee.

Both men and women with paralysis may experience autonomic dysreflexia during sexual activity. This results in an increase in blood pressure and a decrease in heart rate, sweating, and flushing, and a pounding headache. A feeling of impending doom may accompany this. It is not unusual for this to happen during bladder and bowel care, but when it happens during sexual activity, it may be stressful and cause the person involved to stop all such activity. But some people with spinal cord injury report that these sensations actually contribute in a positive way to their sexual experience and mimic the sensation of sexual arousal.

Body Image Issues

Changes in body image are also significant among those with spinal injury. Quadriplegics lose muscle tone, especially in the abdominal area; this is often called "quad belly" and may generate feelings of unattractiveness. Loss of muscle tone and coordination may also affect the ability to hold and caress the sexual partner.

People with spinal cord injury are often intolerant to cold, and being naked poses a problem as they often feel uncomfortable. Their extremities may also feel very cold to the touch; this can affect the sexual partner, who may avoid touching them. It is usual for the person with a spinal cord lesion not to sweat below the level of the injury but to sweat excessively as well as to flush above the level of the injury. This can both feel and look unattractive and may also act as a barrier to being naked with a partner.

These body image issues may be more pronounced for women, and single women with spinal cord injury describe their difficulties in finding a new partner as being directly related to their feelings about themselves, lack of self esteem, and negative feelings about their altered body.

Solutions

There is some evidence that the topic of sexuality in spinal cord injury is not discussed even in the rehabilitation phase. This is a matter of concern, as education is a key component of recovery and without it, many people are left with unanswered questions and uncertainty.

Traditionally, men have been advised to use either the vacuum pump or intracavernosal injections to achieve erections. There are effective, although they are both quite invasive and dropout rates are quite high. They both require manual dexterity, which can be a challenge for those with weakness or paralysis of the upper limbs. This can be solved by having the partner use the pump on the man or give the injection, but this may not be palatable for some partners. For men, the advent of the PDE5 inhibitors Viagra and Levitra has been extremely positive. Both these medications have been shown to be effective in up to 94 percent of men using them, but they are more effective in men with incomplete lesions and in men with higher lesions. Levitra has been shown to also enable men to ejaculate, although the reason why this happens is not clear.

Many women and men report that after the injury, they are able to develop new areas above the level of the lesion that are sensitive and lead to arousal and perhaps even orgasm. Exploration of this phenomenon should be encouraged, as some may find themselves able to achieve orgasm through stimulation of these erogenous zones.

Women with spinal cord injury may be more likely to have an orgasm if they use a vibrator, as the intensity of stimulation is much higher than with manual or oral stimulation. This is also helpful to the sexual partner, who may become fatigued with oral or manual stimulation only and may also develop sexual problems in response to the lack of responsivity of the person with the spinal cord injury.

CONCLUSION

Injury from trauma is unfortunately a reality of modern life. Young people experience traumatic injury in far greater numbers than the older population. Men are more likely than women to suffer a traumatic spinal or head injury. Many of these injuries are severe, with lifelong consequences, including sexual difficulties.

WEB SITES

http://www.paralinks.net/sexualitysci.html
This Web site contains a long list of resources for people with spinal cord injury on the topic of sexuality. There are fact sheets for men and women on the topic as well as links to organizations and university centers that have research programs in this field.

http://www.ahrq.gov/clinic/tp/sexlsptp.htm
This is a link to the AHRQ (Agency for Healthcare Research and Quality) Web site and its report on spinal cord injury and sexuality. The AHRQ provides evidence-based reports on many different health topics.

http://www.sexualhealth.com/channel.php?Action=view_sub&channel=3&topic=11
The Sexual Health Network maintains this Web site, on which questions and answers about sexuality after spinal cord injury are presented.

Chapter Nine

SEXUALITY IN MEN WITH CANCER

All of those who experience a cancer diagnosis and then go through treatment will experience either short-term or permanent alterations to their sexual lives. Cancers that are unique to men present challenges, as these cancers directly affect male sexual functioning. In this chapter, cancer of the prostate, penis, and testicle will be described, along with the sexual side effects and solutions to these problems.

PROSTATE CANCER

Prostate cancer is the most frequently diagnosed cancer in men and also the leading cause of cancer deaths. But if it is diagnosed and treated early, 100 percent of men will survive this cancer. Prostate cancer usually occurs in men over the age of 60, and seldom occurs before age 45. There are few suspicious signs of this disease but if there are, they include changes in urinary function (frequent need to urinate, urinating frequently at night, weak stream, and difficulty starting to urinate). A more common finding is an abnormal digital rectal exam and raised prostate-specific antigen (PSA) in the blood. Most prostate cancers today are detected as a result of PSA screening. A biopsy of the prostate is usually performed to make the diagnosis.

Bob is 62 years old and a manager at a large power company in the Midwest. He went for his annual physical last year and was surprised to learn that his PSA (prostate-specific antigen) test had risen. He was referred to a urologist and a biopsy of his prostate was performed. Two weeks later, he heard the words he'd been dreading: you have prostate cancer. Bob had recently married for the second time, and his wife Betty was devastated by the news.

Treatment of prostate cancer is usually successful, and most men go on to live out their lives and die of something else. But the treatments for this kind of cancer have a significant impact on quality of life, especially in the sexual domain. The most common treatment for this cancer is *radical prostatectomy*. In this surgery, the prostate and seminal vesicles are removed through one incision in the abdomen or a number of smaller incisions if the surgery is done either by laparoscopic or robotic technique. The two major side effects of this treatment are erectile dysfunction (ED) and urinary incontinence.

In the 1980s, an urologist named Patrick Walsh pioneered a new surgical technique for this surgery. Using this technique, the nerve bundles that run on the outside of the prostate gland, one on each side, are preserved and not destroyed when the prostate gland is removed. Depending on the amount of cancer in the prostate, one or both of these nerve bundles may be spared. These are the nerves that are responsible for erections, and the damage to them in dictates in part how good or bad the man's erections will be after the surgery. The other factor that is really important is the health of the penile tissue itself; lack of blood flow and oxygen resulting from the absence of erections can further impact on the man's ability to regain erections after the surgery. Due to the average age of men who are diagnosed with this cancer (60 to 70 years), some men may already be experiencing changes in their erections before the diagnosis, and any treatment tends to make these worse.

The surgery went well, and Bob was surprised that he had so little pain. Betty had taken three weeks off work to look after him, but after the first 10 days or so, it was obvious that he was doing well and didn't need all that much looking after. After two weeks, the catheter was taken out, and when he went for his post-op appointment with the urologist, he was pleased to learn that the cancer was contained in the prostate and that he had every hope for a complete cure.

But as the weeks and months went by, Bob was growing increasingly frustrated by the lack of erectile response he was experiencing. The urologist had said he had been able to spare the nerves, so why was Bob not having any erections? He tried to stimulate himself, and Betty tried to stimulate him, too. But nothing was happening down there.

Men who have both nerve bundles spared during surgery stand a better chance of regaining erections after the surgery. It is also better if one nerve bundle is spared than if both are destroyed during the surgery. Between 30 percent and 85 percent of men who have both nerve bundles spared will eventually regain the ability to have an erection that is firm enough for penetration. But these erections may still not last long enough to satisfy both partners, and they also may not be reliable. Most men will need some form of erectile aid to achieve erections following the surgery. Even when the nerve bundles are saved, damage is caused during the surgery by surgical instruments and the heat from the cautery that is used to stop the bleeding; and inflammation may result from the trauma of the surgery.

As many as 70 percent of men will also notice that their penis is shorter in length and smaller in girth following radical prostatectomy. This often comes as a surprise, as many men are not warned that this can happen. It is probably due to early changes in the penile tissue from nerve damage in the first three to six months after the surgery.

Recovery of erections is dependent on age (younger men have greater success), erectile function before the surgery, the size of the prostate gland (smaller size means better outcomes), and the surgical technique used. Problems with erections can continue for years after the surgery, but improvement may be seen up to five years later.

> Bob had read all the books from the library about prostate cancer. He even went to the local support group meetings, but it seemed as if no one wanted to talk about problems with erections. He and Betty had stopped talking about it too. She said it didn't matter to her, but he knew otherwise. They had only been married for just over a year, and before this cancer, things had been great. He knew it was probably just the newness of it all, but he had really enjoyed having regular sex again, and Betty seemed to enjoy it too. At least she said she did.

Erectile difficulties cause a lot of bother for men, and their quality of life suffers. This also impacts on their self-confidence, masculinity, and self-esteem. Some men become withdrawn, and social relationships may change as a result. But some men take this in their stride; they beat the cancer and that is enough for them. For the man who was having erectile difficulties before the cancer, it may not be a big deal.

Because the seminal vesicles are removed during the surgery, the man will no longer experience ejaculation with orgasm. The lack of emission may alter the sensation of orgasm for some men. Orgasm is still possible for men after surgery for prostate cancer. And orgasms still occur even without an erection. This comes as a surprise to some men who were not told about it before the surgery. But most men state that it is a pleasant surprise! Orgasms may be more or less pleasurable than before, and some men will experience pain with orgasm. This is more common in the months following the surgery and usually disappears in time.

> Almost exactly a year after the surgery, Bob noticed that he had a half erection in the shower. He couldn't believe his eyes! He even called Betty to see it. It happened the next day too, and the next. So Bob invited Betty into the shower with him. It was

not enough for penetration, but with good stimulation he could have an orgasm, and this delighted both of them.

Just when things seemed to be improving, however, something else cropped up. He noticed that when he or Betty stimulated his penis, he would have some leakage of urine. He leaked at other times too, but this was just too much. The first time it happened, Betty pulled her hand away quickly and he saw the look on her face.

The other major side effect of prostate surgery that can affect sexual functioning is urinary incontinence. During the surgery to remove the prostate gland, one of the valves (or sphincters) is usually damaged or destroyed. This causes difficulties in controlling the bladder, and many men will have some degree of leakage in the days, weeks, months, or years following the surgery. Some men notice that they have some leakage of urine when they become even partially aroused, and others report leakage during intercourse. This can be bothersome to both the man and his partner, even though urine is sterile and won't harm anyone. Bed linens can be protected by a rubber or plastic sheet, and if the leakage is minimal, a strategically placed towel may be sufficient. But this leakage may be bothersome enough that some men avoid sexual activity out of fear that it will happen.

Another common and effective treatment for prostate cancer is *radiation therapy*. This may be given externally (external beam radiation; EBRT) or internally through the placement of numerous radioactive seeds directly into the prostate (brachytherapy). The amount of erectile difficulty that occurs after this kind of treatment is dependent in part on the type of radiation, with up to 84 percent of men experiencing some changes in their erections. Why these changes occur is less clear than in the case of surgery. It is thought that damage to blood vessels from the radiation may play a role; blood supply and oxygen is reduced and the penis itself becomes less responsive. Radiation to the bulb of the penis, which is inside the body, may also play a role. In the case of brachytherapy, the insertion of needles in order to place the radioactive seeds may cause some internal physical damage affecting erections.

Unlike the situation following surgery, when there is an immediate loss of erections and improvement over time, following radiation therapy, erectile problems seem to occur starting 12 months after the treatment. At the two-year mark, whatever erections the man is having tend to be as good or as bad as they will get. Three years after external beam radiation, 50 percent of men will experience some degree of ED. Men who have brachytherapy tend to have fewer erectile problems and are generally satisfied with their level of functioning three years after treatment. Men with more advanced prostate cancer may receive a combination of brachytherapy and EBRT, and this increases the risk for ED. If they also need to have androgen ablation treatment, their erectile functioning becomes even worse. Following any form of radiation treatment to the prostate, the amount of ejaculate decreases and may disappear completely. But men should not assume that they are sterile, as there have been reports of men fathering children following brachytherapy.

Cryosurgery is another treatment for prostate cancer, in which the prostate tissue and the cancer are frozen and the cancer is hopefully destroyed. The side effects of this procedure include urinary incontinence, perineal pain, destruction of the tissue in the urethra, and ED, but with improvements in the technology, these are much less common than before. The impact on erections is significant, with less than 20 percent of men who have this procedure regaining erections three years after the treatment. For this reason, it is usually offered to men who already have problems with erections or who state that erections are not important to them.

Men who are diagnosed with advanced prostate cancer are generally treated with medications to suppress testosterone production. This is called *androgen deprivation therapy;* it is sometimes called "hormone therapy," although this is not an accurate description of what occurs. Lack of testosterone slows down the growth of the cancer, which needs testosterone to grow. In the past, men were given estrogen, which had the same effect, or had their testicles removed. Surgical removal of the testicles (orchiectomy) leads to an immediate cessation of testosterone production. This procedure is sometimes offered and accepted instead of the injections, which are expensive and require repeated medical visits. But the thought of losing their testicles can be very distressing to some men, and this treatment has fallen out of favor in recent years. These treatments are rarely used today because another treatment (injectable luteinizing hormone-releasing hormone [LHRH] agonists) has been developed, which interrupts the message from the brain to the testicles, causing the testicles to stop producing the male hormone. There is also another drug, a nonsteroidal antiandrogen, which interferes with any testosterone in the blood, reducing the amount of testosterone that can feed the cancer. This is usually used in addition to the injections for a period of time and not as primary treatment, as it is more effective to shut down the production of testosterone.

Androgen deprivation therapy has far-reaching effects on all aspects of sexual functioning. Men describe changes in body image and in the way they perceive themselves as men. They also report changes in their spousal relationships. The lack of testosterone destroys sexual drive or libido. This results in an absence of sexual thoughts, fantasies, and dreams. Men also report that sexual pleasure is no longer possible. Other side effects of this treatment include hot flashes, which can be worse at night, disturbing sleep, an increase in the volume of breast tissue, lack of energy, depression, irritability, and ED. These are extremely bothersome to men and contribute to a lower quality of life while on this type of treatment. Men with low or no desire for sex may experience less distress when they cannot have an erection than men who still desire sex but cannot have an erection. When the medication is stopped, hormone production may resume 18 to 24 weeks later, but some men have to stay on the medication for many years.

Solutions

> Bob makes an appointment to see his urologist after Betty gave him an ultimatum. She told him that if he didn't make the appointment, she would, and she'd go alone to the urologist if she had to. He has been very depressed about the state of his sex life, and it's beginning to cause some problems with Betty. He knows it's his fault, but he just wants to be left alone. He's even stopped hugging and kissing her; what's the point? There's nothing he can do after the hugging and kissing.

Some men may be prepared to live with sexual problems after treatment; they may think that they're lucky to be alive and that being cured of the cancer is the most important thing. This may be the belief of their health care providers as well. Even though there is a range of treatments for erectile dysfunction, men with prostate cancer often do not seek medical help for months or even years. Some men don't remember that they were told about the potential for erectile problems after treatment for prostate cancer. While erections are not necessary for life, and the lack of penetrative intercourse may be more or less important to some couples, lack of sexual activity may impact on the spousal relationship by causing distance between the two partners. Some couples use sex to solve problems, to resolve arguments, or as a means of communication. The absence of intercourse may lead to an absence of touching and a lack of connection and intimacy between the partners. This can cause emotional distress and may lead to relationship breakdown.

> Bob likes the urologist, even though he hasn't seen him since the surgery. He tells the urologist that he hasn't been able to have erections since the surgery and that it's bothering him. He forgets to tell him about the leaking of urine.
>
> The urologist seems to be in a hurry and hands Bob four small blue boxes. He also gives him a booklet and tells him that all the information he needs is in the booklet. He shakes Bob's hand and wishes him well. Within seven minutes, Bob is on his way home.

There are a number of treatments for ED following treatment for prostate cancer. These include oral medication and other treatments including the vacuum pump, the intraurethral pellet, penile injections, and penile implants. Each has benefits and disadvantages; all require a prescription, patient education, and a varied degree of motivation on the part of both the man and his partner. Men who used any of these after surgery are more satisfied with their sex lives than those who did not.

The first line of treatment for erectile difficulties associated with prostate cancer is usually one of the oral medications that have been in existence since

1998. These drugs are called phosphodiesterase-5 [PDE5] inhibitors, with names such as Viagra (sildenafil), Cialis (tadalafil), and Levitra (vardenafil). PDE5 inhibitors cause the relaxation of smooth muscle in the spongy bodies of the penis, allowing blood to enter with sexual stimulation. Most men can take these medications, unless they have had a stroke or heart attack in the previous six months, are on medications for chest pain, have severe blood pressure problems, or are taking alpha-blockers.

> Bob goes home, and he and Betty read the booklet. It explains about erections and gives some reasons why men have problems with erections. There doesn't seem to be much about the effect of prostate cancer and surgery on erections. But the instructions are clear: take one of the blue pills before you want to have sex, wait an hour, and then try. There is a section about side effects, and Bob just glances over these. They decide that they're going to try over the weekend.

Sildenafil (Viagra) is moderately effective in treating ED after prostate surgery, and not surprisingly, if the man has had nerve-sparing surgery and is younger, he is more likely to have a good result from this medication. If both nerve bundles have been spared in men under 55 years of age, 80 percent of them will have an erection firm enough for penetration in more than 50 percent of attempts if they have taken sildenafil. A smaller proportion of older men (45 percent) between the ages of 56 and 65 years with bilateral nerve-sparing surgery will be able to achieve penetration in 50 percent of attempts. This success rate drops to 33 percent in those over 66 years of age, who comprise the vast majority of men with prostate cancer. If only one nerve bundle is spared, the success rate drops (44 percent of men under 55 years of age); and when both nerve bundles have been destroyed, men will not have erections whatever their age or erectile functioning before the surgery.

The side effects include headache, flushing, nasal congestion, and blue-tinted vision. There have been reports of a serious but rare side effect of vision and hearing loss 24 to 36 hours after ingestion of this drug. If a man who has taken this drug notices the sudden onset of vision and/or hearing loss, he should seek emergency medical attention immediately.

Tadalafil (Cialis) is another PDE5 inhibitor. It stays in the bloodstream longer, which allows for more spontaneity. Theoretically, men may be able to respond to sexual stimulation with an erection from 30 minutes after taking a tablet until 36 hours later. The side effects of this particular medication include headache, heartburn, sore muscles, stuffy nose, and back pain. Among men who have had both nerve bundles spared in the surgery, about 50 percent will achieve an erection firm enough for penetration.

The last of this class of drugs is called vardenafil (Levitra); it allows erections faster than the others (in 16 minutes according to one study, as opposed to an hour for the other two drugs). Up to 34 percent of men who have had one or both nerve bundles spared during surgery respond to this particular drug. The short period between taking the drug and being able to have an erection may allow for more spontaneity and may be preferred by couples. Men who have had radiation therapy and then experience erectile difficulties also respond to these drugs. But over time they appear to respond less well.

> The next weekend, Bob and Betty plan to spend Saturday afternoon on this "project." They turn the ringer of the phone off and make sure the front door is locked. Betty has even purchased a new negligee for the occasion. Bob takes the blue pill after a light lunch and watches some golf on the TV while he waits for the hour to pass. He falls asleep for a few minutes, but Betty wakes him and takes his hand, pulling him toward the bedroom with a smile on her face.
>
> For the next 30 minutes, they dedicate themselves to making something happen. Betty looks lovely in the new negligee and she is wearing a perfume that he loves. But nothing happens. And he soon develops a headache the likes of which he has never experienced before. Betty brings him some pills for that, and he eventually falls asleep. He wakes about two hours later, the headache now just a dull throb behind his eyes. But the disappointment cannot be cured, and once again he feels hopeless.

The oral medications are preferred because they are easy to use and they are not invasive. So why do so many men use these drugs once or twice and then, if they are not successful, stop using them and decide not to try anything else? Some men may do this if the erection they have is not as firm or does not last as long as they would like. Other men may find the cost prohibitive or may not want to go to a doctor for a prescription or refill. Or it may be that their partner is not interested in sex and does not support their use of the drugs or refuses to have sex with them. Many men stop trying if their first or second pill does not result in an erection. But it may take up to eight separate attempts before they have an erection sufficient for penetration. Some men also place a lot of pressure on themselves when taking these medications. They want to be successful and yet a little bit of doubt creeps in, which makes success impossible. Taking the medication alone and then masturbating may lead to success initially, and this gives a man confidence that it will work when he is with his partner. A number of other treatments are under investigation, including a form of alprostadil in a cream format that could be rubbed onto the penis as well as tablets containing phentolamine and apomorphine.

> Bob is depressed that the blue pill didn't work. Betty encourages him to seek help again; she hates to see him so depressed. This time Bob goes to see his family physician. He has known Dr. Kay for many years and they are about the same age. Dr. Kay says he really doesn't specialize in these sorts of things, and suggests that Bob see a sexual medicine specialist. Bob is a little tired of all this running around from one doctor to another, but he is willing to try anything at this point and agrees to the referral.

Three weeks later he sees Dr. Macintosh, the sexual medicine specialist. He is a little surprised to see that she is a woman, but he is getting desperate. Dr. Macintosh takes a long and detailed case history from Bob and then tells him that there are plenty of other things that he can try. He is so happy to hear this that he almost hugs her. She suggests that he try the injection; she has found that this is very effective for men after prostate cancer surgery.

If the man cannot take the above-mentioned drugs or they do not work, alternatives exist. These are usually more mechanical or invasive and include the vacuum constriction device (pump), intraurethral prostaglandin pellets, or penile injections of alprostadil or other medications. A permanent surgical implant is also available. After surgery, a graduated treatment plan is usually suggested, starting with an oral medication as described above and then moving to the vacuum pump, and then to the intraurethral pellet or penile injections. The last treatment to be tried is usually the surgical implant. Even with this graduated approach, less than 20 percent of men will still be using any of these methods one year after starting treatment for ED. Either men don't like the more mechanical nature of achieving erections and so stop trying, or all of these methods fail and the men just give up.

The vacuum pump consists of a hard plastic tube with a hand pump attached. The pump withdraws the air from the tube. and when the lubricated penis is placed in the tube and the pump is activated, blood is drawn into the penis. This causes an erection quite quickly, usually in about two minutes. A special rubber constriction band is placed at the base of the penis to trap the blood in the penis. This band can remain in place only for up to 30 minutes, because while it is in place, the circulation of blood in the penis is limited. The use of this device requires some manual dexterity and may decrease spontaneity, but many couples are able to incorporate it into their sex play and are successful with this. The side effects include bruising of the penis, pain at the site of the elastic band, and decreased sensation for the man, as well as the sensation of a cold penis for the partner. This treatment may be used in conjunction with the oral medications if the man is able to have an erection but not able to maintain it for any length of time.

Intraurethral pellets (MUSE) may help some men have an erection, with success rates between 29 percent and 55 percent. A small pellet (about the size of a grain of rice) containing the medication alprostadil is inserted into the urethra by a special applicator. The penis then needs to be rubbed to disperse the medication, and after about 30 minutes some response should be observed. This medication allows the blood vessels in the spongy tissue to relax and fill with blood. The side effects include pain and burning in the urethra at the place where the medication has been absorbed.

Penile injections involve the introduction of a small amount of medication into the side of the penis via a small needle similar to those used by diabetics for insulin. This is an effective way of causing erections and is particularly effective for men who cannot take the oral medication or do not respond to it. It works like the intraurethral pellet: the spongy tissues fill with blood when the blood vessels relax. Many men find the idea of sticking a needle into their penis challenging and usually require a great deal of support and teaching before they are able to do it. The most significant side effect of this is a prolonged erection (priapism). This can be quite painful and may damage the tissues of the penis if it is not treated. Men who have an erection lasting longer than three to four hours should seek emergency medical treatment. Other more minor side effects include pain at the injection site, bruising, and scarring. Scarring is more likely to occur if the injection is given in the same place repeatedly. Care should be taken to rotate injection sites, and the injection should not be used more than once in a 24-hour period.

Penile implants are generally the last treatment choice for men with ED after prostate cancer. Implants are very effective but not commonly used, due to expense and the fact that they require surgery in order to be placed in the penis. There are different kinds of implant devices; the semi-rigid models require the man to bend the device for intercourse and then bend it again to return it to its usual position. The semi-rigid model results in a partial erection that is often visible even when the man is dressed, but it contains few moving parts and is less likely to malfunction. Inflatable devices are also available. These consist of two cylinders that are implanted along the length of the penis, one on each side. They are connected to a small pump that is placed in the scrotum and is connected to a reservoir containing saline, which is implanted in the abdomen. When an erection is desired, the man pumps the small device in his scrotum. and saline from the reservoir flows into the cylinders, causing an erection. When he no longer wants the erection, the flow of saline is reversed when he once again activates the pump in the scrotum.

Bob is eager to try the injection, but the doctor wants him to talk to Betty about it first. He will need to have a test dose of the injection, and the doctor wants him first to talk to his wife and then to come back to her office for another appointment. He is quite irritated with this but agrees. At least there is some hope!

He tells Betty about the injection, but she seems less than keen. He's a little surprised by this, but she assures him that it's just something she has about needles, and as long as she doesn't have to give him the injection, she'll be okay. Bob is shocked to hear this; it was his plan that she would give the injection! Now he realizes why Dr. Macintosh wanted him to talk to his wife.

Three weeks later, the two of them go to see Dr. Macintosh. She explains how the injection works and shows them how to draw up the medication. She then demonstrates this on Bob, who is really embarrassed that this woman is injecting something into his penis. But his embarrassment quickly goes away when his penis starts to grow. He and Betty laugh in relief; something has worked!

For the last few years, urologists have been using an interesting protocol to optimize erectile functioning after surgery. This is called erectile or penile rehabilitation. The protocol involves the man taking a nightly low dose of sildenafil (Viagra) for months after surgery. This improves the chances that spontaneous erections will return, to a point far beyond what is expected if the man does nothing. An alternative method is for the man to take a full dose of the drug three times a week, with the aim of achieving at least 60 percent rigidity with genital stimulation. The man does not need to have intercourse or even an orgasm; it is the erection that counts, as this brings blood and oxygen to the tissues of the penis. If he is not able to have a 60 percent erection with the drug, then another strategy may be needed. This may include the use of penile injections three times a week.

All forms of penile rehabilitation require high motivation and may be expensive. They also need to be continued for many months, sometimes with no visible success to increase compliance or motivation to continue. These protocols also require specialized teaching and ongoing monitoring and appointments with the urologist or sexual medicine specialist.

Couples counseling may be useful in treating sexual problems following prostate cancer. Men with prostate cancer often receive written information about erectile functioning, but this information tends to be generic and overly optimistic, and it may not answer the specific questions or concerns of the man and his partner. Much patient education material is produced with the financial support of the pharmaceutical industry; it may be biased in favor of one particular drug and may not offer a balanced view for the patient.

Communication is a central aspect of dealing with sexual changes. These changes may lead to long-term difficulties that can impact negatively on a relationship. Some women may not encourage their male partners to find help with erectile problems. This may be a reflection of the woman's level of sexual interest and her view that sex is not important or that it is no longer necessary for the relationship. Couples often don't talk about sensitive topics, in case this upsets one of them. Failure to talk about issues leads to isolation and distancing and may further increase the distress that these couples experience.

Couples counseling can really help people who are struggling with poor communication or changes in their sex life. The presence of a third person, a professional, may be the catalyst that the couple needs in order to talk about this topic. Couples counseling provides an opportunity for dialogue in a nonthreatening atmosphere where gentle prompting from the therapist/counselor facilitates meaningful talking without a relapse into poor communication patterns.

While talking can be helpful for some couples, it will not solve the basic problem of the loss of erections. Many couples miss their usual sexual activities. Some couples do manage to adapt to sexual changes including ED and lack of ejaculation. Many women are satisfied as long as their partner is affectionate and is open to hugging and kissing. But men may be less satisfied with these forms of affection; they may want penetrative intercourse and they may be dissatisfied with anything else.

CANCER OF THE PENIS

Penile cancer is very rare in North America, but it is a cancer that is devastating for a man because of the psychological impact of the diagnosis, the resultant body image issues, and the sexual consequences of treatment. This cancer may be diagnosed late, because commonly something on the skin of the penis is ignored when it first appears. Some men also avoid seeking medical attention because they are scared, and so they are diagnosed late in the disease when it has been spread to the lymph nodes.

> Gary had noticed a small patch of white tissue on his penis some months ago but he thought it was probably dry skin and so he ignored it. It didn't go away, and in fact it seemed to get bigger over time. He had to go the doctor to get his blood pressure checked, and he mentioned it. He was surprised when the doctor looked at it and said that it looked suspicious. Right then and there, the doctor took a scraping from the area, and a week later Gary learned that he had penile cancer.

In the past, this cancer was usually treated with surgical removal of all or part of the penis. More recently treatment has been carried out with a laser, which may spare the tissue of the penis. This cancer has a high recurrence rate, so it is important to remove as much tissue as possible to ensure that the cancer is eradicated; this often means that the surgery is quite extensive and mutilating. Some men also require radiation and/or chemotherapy, depending on the stage and spread of the cancer.

Sexual Changes after Treatment

> Gary was lucky in that the surgeon was able to save part of his penis; he would still be able to pass urine normally, but he was not sure that he would ever have sex again. Gary felt enormous guilt for leaving the situation to go on as long as it had done before seeking medical attention. He was depressed after the surgery and withdrew from his friends and family. Even his wife couldn't reach him. She tried everything she could think of; she cooked him his favorite meals, and one night she even tried to seduce him. He just shook his head and went to watch TV, leaving her alone in the bedroom in tears.

If the whole penis is removed (this is called a penectomy), the man will obviously be unable to have penetrative intercourse. But he may be able to experience pleasurable sensation if the scrotum, upper thighs, and penile stub are stimulated. If only part of the penis is removed, physical shortening of the penis will occur. The man may be able to have penetrative intercourse, and many men are as satisfied with their sex life after this surgery as they were before.

When the glans (or head) of the penis is removed, men may find that intercourse is painful and their partners may also experience pain. It is thought that the head of the penis performs a protective function and acts as a shock absorber during penetrative intercourse. When the head of the penis is missing, pressure is placed on the shaft and the spongy tissue inside the shaft, and this causes pain.

The impact of this cancer and its treatment include alterations to body image and masculinity. Some men may feel ashamed about the size of their penis, but studies show that most men do continue to have sexual activity, even though their interest in sex may decrease somewhat and the frequency of activity may also be reduced. Some may regret their choice of treatment in the light of the sexual consequences and may wish they had chosen less radical surgery. Most men find that if their partner is supportive, sexual interest and satisfaction are regained after treatment.

Solutions

An important part of dealing with the consequences of diagnosing and treating penile cancer is preparing the man and his partner for what lies ahead. Some men may assume that their sex life is over after the surgery. But this is not entirely true; nerves in the genital area usually remain intact even after the removal of the entire penis, and so the man may be responsive to stimulation and may even experience the sensation of orgasm when appropriate areas are touched. Alternatives to penetrative intercourse (such as heavy petting) are always possible, and the man can still provide pleasure to his partner and in turn receive pleasure. It may also be helpful for the couple to use sensate focus exercises). The goal of these exercises is for the man to learn new forms of sensual touch that may open an entirely new sexual repertoire for the couple. This may then encourage the continuation of a meaningful if altered range of sexual activities.

CANCER OF THE TESTICLE

Testicular cancer primarily affects young men at the peak of their sexual lives and may have a profound impact on fertility and masculinity. Many young men find a lump in a testicle in the shower or during sexual activity. Some become so scared that they do not seek medical treatment immediately. But if this cancer is diagnosed and treated early, the prognosis is good. There can be a great deal of shame and embarrassment associated with this cancer, but there are some outstanding advocates, for example Lance Armstrong, who have made this cancer much less stigmatized.

> Bruce was a typical 23-year-old university student. He loved football and baseball and still rollerbladed to his part-time job whenever he could. He had a large group of friends, both male and female, and they enjoyed camping in the summer and went on a yearly ski trip to Colorado. Last year, he felt something in one of his testicles when he was showering. He didn't think much of it, but the next morning it was still there and he thought he had better get it checked out. He went to see the doctor at the student health center and was shocked to hear that he probably had testicular cancer. Within three days he was seen by an urologist and a date was set for surgery to remove the testicle. How could this happen?

Treatment includes surgical removal of the affected testicle; this has the potential to create both immediate and long-range feelings in the patient of being less of a man and being sexually unattractive. Some men report that when the diagnosis is made, they experience a reflex loss of libido. There is no physical cause for this, but the psychological impact can be significant and may be the source of sexual problems. Further treatment may be recommended, based on the grade of the cancer; radiation and/or chemotherapy may be necessary, and these can affect sexual functioning as well as fertility.

Sexual Side Effects of Treatment

> Bruce was lucky; the cancer had not spread and he needed no further treatment. For a while after the surgery, he was really tired and he had to miss the rest of the semester, which frustrated him. His mom came to stay with him for a couple of weeks after the surgery, and she cooked his favorite meals and did his laundry, and for a while he felt as if he was back at home. But she had to go back to work and he needed to get on with things.
> That was easier said than done. He was really unsure of how to act around his friends. They had all visited him in hospital and at his apartment, but things were different with them. They treated him as if he was different and the easy joking between them was gone.

Even though there is no physical cause of changes in sexual functioning after the removal of a testicle, men report a loss of interest in sex as well as changes with regard to orgasm. There is likely a psychological component to these changes. The loss of one testicle does not reduce the levels of testosterone in the body, as the other testicle will still make enough for normal functioning. But if more extensive surgery needs to be done, to remove lymph nodes, for example, the effects on ejaculation may be more pronounced, with men experiencing dry orgasm (no emission). This has a very real impact on fertility.

Radiation treatment effects erectile functioning; men may have fewer erections upon awakening from sleep, and the erections may be less firm than is necessary for penetration and may not last long enough for successful intercourse. Men who have experienced radiation treatment also notice a reduced quantity of ejaculate. Chemotherapy has the most profound effect on sexual functioning, with 25 to 33 percent of men experiencing loss of libido, problems with orgasm and ejaculation, and a decrease in sexual activity. These problems may be expected while chemotherapy is being given, but they seem to persist for as long as six months after treatment is over. When radiation and chemotherapy treatments are combined, the sexual side effects are worse. Men who are older also seem to have worse side effects.

While most men who have been treated for testicular cancer report a decrease in sexual satisfaction, they also report that their relationship with their partner is strengthened.

> Six months later, Bruce was feeling much better. His energy was back, and socially things had improved a lot. He'd met someone when he first went back to his part-time job and now he and Jen were a couple. They'd even changed their Facebook profiles from "single" to "attached." Things were serious between them; cancer had made him realize that life is really precious and you have to live every day to its fullest. But there was this nagging doubt in his head. . . . What if he couldn't have kids? Would it be fair to stay with Jen under those circumstances?

Fertility issues are important for men with testicular cancer. This cancer is most common in young men; they may not be partnered and so may not be thinking about having children; or they may be newly partnered and this diagnosis comes at a time when they are planning to have children. What is interesting is that 75 percent of men who are diagnosed with testicular cancer have decreased sperm production at the time of diagnosis. This is thought to be associated with an undescended testicle or testicles, which alters fertility. Some men may be able to father a child naturally, but most will require some form of assistance from a fertility specialist.

> Bruce talked to his oncologist about this, and he was sent to see a fertility specialist. He was very nervous about the appointment, because he didn't know what to expect. The fertility specialist was an older man who had a rather gruff manner; he was very matter-of-fact about Bruce's chances of being able to father a baby and suggested that Bruce have a sperm count. Bruce had heard stories about this and was very embarrassed when a young woman directed him to a small room with a TV and a pile of magazines and handed him a small plastic cup. It took him a while but he managed to do what he had to and produced a sperm sample.
> A few days later he received a call from the fertility clinic. His sperm count was on the low side of normal, and the clinic representative suggested that at the time when

he wanted to have children with someone, he and his partner should come back to the clinic for further testing and perhaps even some immediate help. Bruce was not sure what to make of this information. Did he have enough sperm or didn't he?

Men who are young, unmarried, and childless experience more infertility-related distress than those who have fathered children and are in a supportive relationship. The diagnosis is often a time of great crisis, and some men may refuse to have their sperm frozen. Months or years later, when they are in a relationship, they may regret not banking their sperm. Younger men may not have the opportunity to consider and discuss loss of fertility or may find it difficult to discuss it with their parents or health care providers. In the case of men under the age of 18 years, the decision may have to be made by the parents, who may be very distraught and unable to think of anything but their son's survival; they may not even consider his future fertility. It may be very embarrassing for the parent or parents even to suggest sperm banking, but this is an important topic and hopefully, the health care team will discuss it with both the young man and his parents.

> Bruce thought about his low sperm count over the next few weeks and this led him to thinking about the time when he was diagnosed. Why had no one suggested that he bank his sperm before his testicle was removed? He could not get these thoughts out of his mind. Over the next few days he grew angry, remembering the speed with which he had had his surgery. He couldn't even remember anyone talking to him about sperm banking.

It is suggested that *all* men diagnosed with testicular cancer should bank sperm in case they need to use it at some time in the future. This banking can be done in just a few days before any treatment is started. Adequate sperm samples can be collected with only 24 to 48 hours between collections, and new in vitro fertilization techniques offer increased success. This is a very difficult but very important topic for a young man who is not in a relationship.

> Bruce found himself avoiding his old friends. He and Jen were fighting a lot, too. He was just so angry all the time and even though he was not angry with her, Jen felt that his anger was misplaced. She told him over and over again that the loss of his testicle did not mean he was any different from any other guy, but he didn't agree. He was different; anyone could see that. And then Jen left; she just couldn't get through to him and so she left.

A diagnosis of testicular cancer carries with it some unique social and cultural challenges. Body image and masculinity are profoundly impacted by this cancer. For many, the testicles are a symbol of masculinity and an outward sign of being a "normal" man. Being a normal man is associated with being able to perform sexually. The loss of a testicle threatens all this, and the cancer is a threat to life itself. Some men who have had a testicle removed have some body image problems; they may be distressed about what has happened to their body and feel unattractive. They may be reluctant to undress in front of other men in the locker room or may feel embarrassed using a public urinal.

Solutions

A significant element in the sexual difficulties for these men is the effect of the treatment on body image. Many men are not aware that an artificial testicle can be implanted in the scrotum after treatment is complete. This allows the man to look like he did before the surgery and does much to improve his body image and confidence. Most men who have had such an implant see a significant improvement in their sexual self-esteem after the intervention.

Intimate relationships tend to be strengthened by the cancer; partners are usually very supportive, and a challenge like this can draw couples closer together. Relationship distress is more likely to occur in newly partnered couples. Some women find that during the treatment phase they take on a more maternal role in contrast to the expected role of sexual partner; this can be challenging to the balance in the partnership. Men often become quite isolated during treatment and do not communicate their thoughts and feelings to their partner. This can cause distancing and emotional distress.

Erectile difficulties may be caused by nerve and blood vessel damage; the oral medications used to treat ED may help, but if the issue is mostly psychological, they may not be that effective. Problems with ejaculation are more difficult to treat. Preparation for any changes should be an essential component of any treatment plan. Many men do not anticipate that they will have problems if they are not discussed, and so when problems occur, they do not seek help but suffer in silence.

CONCLUSION

The cancers affecting only men pose direct and significant challenges to sexual functioning, primarily because the sexual organs are affected. While medication is available to treat erectile dysfunction, it is not always effective. and many men suffer emotionally because of the changes due to cancer and its treatments.

SUGGESTED READING

Alterowitz, R., and B. Alterowitz. *Intimacy with Impotence: The Couple's Guide to Better Sex after Prostate Cancer.* Cambridge, MS: Da Capo Lifelong Books, 2004.

Katz, A. *Breaking the Silence on Cancer and Sexuality: A Handbook for Health Care Providers.* Pittsburgh, PA: Oncology Nursing Society, 2007.

Katz, A. *Woman Cancer Sex.* Pittsburgh, PA: Oncology Nursing Society, 2009.

Laken, V., and K. Laken. *Making Love Again.* East Sandwich, MS: North Star Publications, 2002.

Perlman, G., and J. Drescher. *A Gay Man's Guide to Prostate Cancer.* New York: Haworth Press, 2005.

Schover, L. *Sexuality and Fertility after Cancer.* New York: John Wiley & Sons, 1997.

WEB SITES

http://www.mdanderson.org/topics/sexuality/

This Web site is from M. D. Anderson Cancer Center at the University of Texas. It contains a wealth of important information for men, women, and adolescents, with videos and text.

http://www.cancer.org/docroot/MIT/MIT_7_1x_SexualityforMenandTheirPartners.asp?sitearea=&level=

This Web site is presented by the American Cancer Society and includes a variety of different topics for men with cancer and their partners.

www.fertilehope.org

Fertile Hope is a national nonprofit organization dedicated to providing reproductive information, support, and hope to cancer patients and survivors whose medical treatments present the risk of infertility.

www.planetcancer.org

This Web site is targeted at young adults with cancer. It contains information for this population that is presented with irony and humor.

www.seankimerling.org

This Web site promotes testicular self-examination and seeks to provide information about testicular cancer.

http://www.ulmanfund.org/Default.aspx

This is another Web site designed for young adults with cancer.

Chapter Ten

SEXUALITY IN WOMEN WITH CANCER

The cancers that affect women include breast cancer and the gynecological cancers including cancer of the cervix, vulva, and vagina. These cancers, reproductive and sexual organs and their treatment causes long-term physical and emotional consequences. Central to this is the impact of surgery, radiation, and chemotherapy on body image, which plays a large role in terms of how women see themselves as sexual beings.

BREAST CANCER

Breast cancer is the most commonly diagnosed cancer and the second most common cause of cancer death in women. Ninety-eight percent of women with breast cancer that has not spread will survive this disease. This means that there are many women today who have had breast cancer and have gone on to lead otherwise normal lives. But the sequelae of treatment persist for years, and these include sexual problems.

> Diane is 47 years old and a teacher with three grown sons. Last year, she was diagnosed with breast cancer after a routine mammogram. She was shocked when she received the call from her family nurse practitioner and was soon in the emotionally turbulent situation of having to make a decision about what treatment to have. She was just overwhelmed and scared and didn't know where to turn. The nurse practitioner was really helpful and spent a lot of time talking to her and explaining the different options, but everything was still confusing. Eventually she just told the surgeon to do what he thought was best and she would live with the consequences.

Breast cancer is treated according to stage as well as whether certain receptors are present in the cancer. Early breast cancer can be treated by *breast conserving surgery* (lumpectomy, partial mastectomy, segmental resection, or quadrectomy) followed by radiation therapy. Some women require more extensive surgery (*radical mastectomy*), in which all the breast tissue is removed. It is not uncommon for women to opt for this surgery even if their cancer is diagnosed early; they may feel more confident that all the cancer is gone if all the breast tissue is removed. Many women have reconstruction of the breast either at the time of the surgery or some time after the surgery. There are a variety of ways of doing this, including the use of skin and fat from the stomach to create a new breast or the use of saline or silicone implants.

> Diane had the affected breast removed. She recovered quite quickly from the surgery and soon resumed her regular activities. Six weeks after surgery, she started chemotherapy. She was not looking forward to this, as she had heard so many stories about how awful it was. And she didn't look forward to losing her hair. But she knew she was strong and she knew she could cope.
>
> What she didn't expect was the way the loss of her breast would affect how she felt about herself. Since the surgery she'd been unable even to look at herself in the mirror. The only time she'd seen the scar was the day the bandages came off and the sight of the red scar across her chest had made her gasp. Since then she'd not looked. She closed her eyes when she dried herself after her shower. She kept her eyes closed when she hastily fastened her bra and shoved the little bag of foam into the cup on that side.
>
> No one knew about this; she hadn't even talked to Brent, her husband, about it. She dressed and undressed in the bathroom now, and he was his usual respectful self and didn't say anything or ask any questions. She felt awful about this but she hadn't worked it out in her own head yet. So how could she talk about it?

Breast cancer survivors report that a major factor impacting on sexuality following treatment is changes to body image. Body image issues may surface at the time when the diagnosis is made. Women have described their breasts as being "medicalized" at this time, when they are poked and prodded by various health care providers. This continues during treatment when the women are cut and/or radiated. Women who have radiation therapy state that in order to get through the daily exposure of their breasts to various personnel in the treatment area, they dissociate from their breasts as sexual organs. This is a coping mechanism and works quite well, but it may become a source of future problems when women remain dissociated from their breasts during sex or no longer see their breasts as sexual organs. Some women also develop swelling of the arm on the affected side if lymph nodes have been removed during surgery. This lymphedema may be seen by women as further impacting on their view of themselves. Many women wear a special sleeve on that arm to reduce or prevent the swelling, and this may be seen as a further reminder of the cancer and also as unattractive.

> Diane's nurse practitioner (NP) called her about two weeks after she'd started chemotherapy. Diane was a little surprised but was glad that the NP cared enough to follow up with her. She agreed to make an appointment, and one week later found herself in the NP's office. All it took was one question: "How are you really feeling?" The floodgates opened and Diane sobbed out her feelings.
>
> The nurse practitioner sat and listened until Diane stopped talking. "It sounds as if your body image has really been affected by this. Have you thought about having reconstructive surgery?" Diane nodded; that had been mentioned by the surgeon, but in the fog of those early days, it just seemed too much. But she hadn't expected to feel this way and maybe having reconstruction would help.
>
> Four weeks later, she saw the plastic surgeon. He examined her and told her that she could have further surgery and that she had a choice between a saline or silicone implant. More decisions! The surgery would be done after she'd finished her chemotherapy, and she was glad that this time she had some time to prepare. She was actually managing the chemotherapy quite well, and even though she hated the wig she was wearing, she knew it wasn't forever and her hair would grow back.
>
> Months later she had the reconstructive surgery. She chose the saline implant and was both excited and nervous about the results. The pain from this surgery was more difficult than from her first surgery. She seemed to hurt more than when her breast was removed. The nurses in the hospital said this was normal, as the skin and muscles had to stretch to accommodate the implant.
>
> When the bandages came off, she was surprised to find herself in tears again. The breast just looked so different! She tried to hide her disappointment and persuaded herself that it would get better. But it didn't. She found herself hating that breast more and more. It looked different and felt different. It was hard and didn't move like her other breast. But she couldn't tell anyone; people would just think she was ungrateful.

Women who have breast-conserving surgery (lumpectomy) and those who have breast reconstruction seem to have a better body image than those who undergo mastectomy. But this does not apply to all women. Even with lumpectomy, the breast may be altered in appearance, and women may be disappointed with this if they expected the breast to look the same as it did before. The area around the scar from the lumpectomy may feel different; the breast may be numb or very sensitive in that area. The presence of a scar can be a permanent reminder of the cancer, and some women never come to terms with this. If the woman has had reconstruction following surgery, the reconstructed breast may also look and feel quite different from the other, unaffected breast, and many women do not expect this. Other issues affecting body image include hair loss from chemotherapy, weight loss or gain, and the response of the partner to these changes.

Hair loss is a common side effect of chemotherapy, and it has a major impact on women's body image. The loss of hair on the head may make women feel unattractive, but the loss of pubic hair can also impact on women's perception of themselves as sexual beings. Many women report that they are very embarrassed by the loss of pubic hair and that this is a barrier to feeling and acting like an adult sexual partner, because in their minds, a naked mons pubis looks like that of a little girl. In addition, some women are not warned that their pubic hair will fall out during chemotherapy, and this loss comes as a shock.

So while surgery to the breast has no direct effect on the anatomy or physiology of the sexual response, it certainly raises issues that relate to sexuality. The partner's response to the altered breast is also important. While many partners are accepting and supportive and tell the woman that she is the same person and she is loved and desired, it is the internal dialogue that the woman has with herself about her desirability and attractiveness that really impacts on her acceptance of herself. Some partners try very hard to pay attention to the affected breast or side of the chest (in the case of mastectomy). This may be a positive thing, but some women say they have altered sensation there and it hurts or feels numb when it is touched, and they don't want to hurt their partner's feelings because he or she is being so kind and trying so hard.

Women who have *radiation therapy* in addition to some form of surgery report that they feel very tired during the course of radiation and this can impact on their desire for sex. Many women continue to shoulder the burden of their work and family commitments during the radiation treatments, and they are just exhausted at the end of every day; sex is the last thing on their mind. It is also quite common for women to develop some skin damage during the course of treatment. This looks and feels like a bad sunburn and makes women sensitive to touch in that area. The tattoo marks that are placed on the skin of the chest wall to guide the radiation treatments may also serve as a constant and permanent reminder of the cancer.

> Diane learned to live with her reconstructed breast. She'd learned to live with every-thing else this disease threw at her. The latest was that she had to take medication for the next five years or more to prevent a recurrence of the cancer. The chemotherapy seemed to have stopped her periods and she was in the throes of menopause. She had hot flashes that woke her at night. During the day, she walked around the house in a T-shirt and shorts and tried her best not to go out anywhere.
>
> Life was just so different now. Even though she knew she was supposed to feel better now that she had the new breast, she still hadn't allowed Brent to see it. Their sex life was a distant memory and they didn't even talk about it. He seemed okay about this; at least he didn't complain any more. They'd tried to make love once, just before she had the second surgery. It had hurt so much that she'd almost screamed; Brent had retreated to his side of the bed and that was the end of that.

The most profound impact on a woman's sexual functioning is from *chemotherapy* and/or hormone-manipulating drugs. Many women who receive chemotherapy as part of the treatment regimen for breast cancer experience changes in various aspects of their sexual responses. This is in part due to the effect of the chemotherapy on the ovaries; the aim of the chemotherapy is to shut off the ovaries' production of estrogen, and the resultant lack of estrogen is what causes the sexual changes. One of these changes is complete disappearance of libido (in 65 percent of women) or a significant lessening of interest in sex (up to 48 percent of women). Women also report vaginal dryness as a result of the lowered estrogen levels. This can lead to pain during, which also contributes to decreased interest in sex or avoidance of sexual activity. Younger women with breast cancer treated with chemotherapy may also experience problems with orgasm, although why this happens is not clear.

The symptoms of ovarian failure are often worse for women who have not yet gone through menopause. Women who are postmenopausal and on some form of hormone therapy for the alleviation of symptoms may have to stop the hormone therapy in order to eradicate any estrogen, and this may bring back their symptoms (such as hot flashes or vaginal dryness).

These sexual changes persist long after the treatment is over; 80 percent of women have reported sexual difficulties five years after treatment. An additional problem is due to the thinning of the tissues of the vagina and vulva; women become more susceptible to urinary tract infections. An extra barrier to a normal sex life is created if intercourse leads to a painful bladder infection.

Chemotherapy may also predispose women to weight gain, which is an important factor in body image. Many women will gain 10 pounds or more in the months and years after treatment, and this may also lead to sexual avoidance.

Diane started taking the medication to prevent a cancer recurrence. This seemed to make her menopausal symptoms much worse. She was now having up to 10 hot flashes a day, and at night they seemed to come even more often. She could barely keep up with the laundry this produced; she had to wash the sheets every day and started sleeping on a large towel, which she changed after each bout of sweating. She wasn't sure how long she could take this. She was irritable and tired from not getting enough sleep. And Brent had started complaining about the lack of sex in their life. Sex? She hadn't thought about that for ages. It was just not a part of her life anymore and he had to deal with that.

Women with breast cancer that is estrogen-receptor positive usually have additional treatment to eradicate any estrogen in their bodies in order to prevent a recurrence of the cancer. One of the more common of these treatments is the drug tamoxifen. This drug lowers estrogen and progesterone and causes symptoms like that of the menopause. Tamoxifen has some effect on the vaginal mucosa and tends to lessen vaginal dryness, and so some women find that it provides some relief from the vaginal dryness experienced as a result of chemotherapy. Many women on this drug report that it decreases their libido significantly. In the past few years, it has been shown that after taking tamoxifen for three to five years, women with estrogen-receptor positive breast cancer receive additional benefit from taking one of the aromatase inhibitors, another group of drugs that have similar estrogen-suppressive side effects including hot flashes and vaginal dryness. It has been noted that some women on these drugs develop such severe vaginal dryness that any kind of vaginal penetration is impossible due to the pain and narrowing of the vagina.

Women who do not have a partner at the time of their diagnosis and treatment have some special needs. The impact of the treatments on body image of may make these women reluctant to pursue a new relationship, out of fear that someone new may reject their altered body. A woman who has a partner may have more confidence in this regard. How and when to disclose that one has had cancer is also a sensitive topic, but not one that is unique to breast cancer survivors. Younger women with breast cancer tend to have more difficulty coping with the diagnosis and are also more likely to report a poorer quality of life and depression. Depression is often treated with a class of drugs called serotonin reuptake inhibitors, which cause problems with libido, arousal, and orgasm, further compounding the side effects of chemotherapy and other treatments.

Solutions

One of the issues in posttreatment adaptation to a changed body is that information tends to be given to women during the decision-making phase after diagnosis. This is a time when most people hear only a small part of what they are told. Information needs to be given all along the treatment journey, so that the woman can hear what she needs at a time when she is most able to hear it.

It's important to deal with the anticipated changes due to treatment before the treatment begins, so that the woman is as well prepared as possible for what lies ahead. With regard to coming to terms with altered body image, women need an accurate idea of what their breasts may look like following lumpectomy, mastectomy, and reconstruction. Showing them photographs of other women who have had any one of these surgical procedures can be helpful. But this is a lot to deal with, especially when women are reeling from the shock of diagnosis. Some women refuse to view photographs and afterward wish they had, as their reaction to their own breast(s) may not be what they expected. Before-and-after photographs can be very helpful in preparing women and their partners and may also be useful in starting the dialogue about sexual changes. For women who are not able to have reconstruction or who do not want reconstruction, seeing and touching the many different kinds of breast prostheses can also be helpful.

When the treatment is over, a woman may need to find a way to reconnect to her body and her image of her body. This may take a long time and much effort. Some women don't find this easy to do; they avoid looking at their altered breast or that part of their chest where their breast once was. They don't allow their partner to see them undressed, and they start changing in the bathroom.

The partner's acceptance of a woman's changed body is also an important part of healing, but if the partner does not have the opportunity to see what has changed, the partner's response may not be helpful. Some partners make a deliberate effort to touch and caress the altered breast, scar, or chest wall. This may be helpful, but some women find that any touching of that area causes pain due to increased sensitivity. The same can be said for touching the breast after radiation therapy, when the skin may be sensitive. If the couple is not able to talk about this openly and honestly, then further problems may arise. The woman must be able to tell her partner what feels good and what doesn't. The partner needs to be able to see her undressed so that his or her perception of what is changed is accurate.

Not all partners find it easy to accept the physical changes that a woman has gone through. The partner's response will directly affect the way the woman feels about herself. Women state that their partner's desire for them in spite of the physical changes is an important part of self-acceptance and self-confidence.

Some women find that physical exercise is an important part of the recovery process and acceptance of the changed body. Any exercise that involves lifting weights should be approved by a physician, as this may impact on the development of swelling in the arm on the affected side if lymph nodes have been removed. Dancing has been shown to improve body image and lift depression.

Perhaps the greatest challenge is for a woman to learn that her body can once again be a source of pleasure instead of pain. Sensate focus exercises can be very helpful in achieving this. These exercises have traditionally been used to help couples reconnect with each other in the face of challenges to sexual functioning. The end goal is usually the resumption of sexual intercourse, but a modified version of the exercises may be helpful for a woman who has had breast cancer and her partner. Traditionally, these exercises include four stages: a modified, two-stage version of the exercises is presented here.

SENSATE FOCUS EXERCISES FOR WOMEN WITH BREAST CANCER

The object of these exercises is to help a woman with breast cancer learn to experience pleasure from her body. The goal is not to have intercourse or an orgasm.

The woman must be allowed to control the pace and extent of the touching, as it is vital that she be comfortable and relaxed throughout the exercise.

All distractions must be controlled: switch off the ringer on the phone, turn off the cell phone and the TV, and lock the door.

This exercise should be done three times a week.

Stay in each of the stages for three weeks before progressing to the next stage.

Each partner takes 10 or 15 minutes to touch the other partner. Guidance about what feels good can be given by the person being touched.

Stage 1: Touch your partner anywhere but the breast area and genitals. You may use massage oil or lotion if desired. You may choose to concentrate your touching on one area (for example, the feet or hands) or to touch all over the body excluding the breasts and genitals.

Stage 2: The breast area may be touched if the woman wants this. She may want only the unaffected breast or side to be touched; that's just fine. She may or may not change her mind next time.

In dealing with the menopausal symptoms associated with treatment, there are a number of medications that may be helpful, as well as some common-sense suggestions to deal with the symptoms. The vasomotor symptoms such as hot flashes can be treated with antidepressants, which have been shown to be effective but have sexual side effects. Clonidine, a medication to lower blood pressure, is effective for some women in halting hot flashes.

The most effective treatment for menopausal symptoms is hormone therapy, but this has not been shown to be safe for women with breast cancer. Local estrogen treatment to the vagina is effective for the treatment of vaginal dryness; however, many women and their oncologists are concerned about the amount of estrogen that gets into the general circulation, even if it is very low. Many of the so-called natural products advertised for the relief of menopausal symptoms are not considered safe for women with breast cancer. Black cohosh and soy products are all phyto-estrogens and may expose women to small amounts of estrogen, which may be too risky. There is also only weak evidence that they provide any relief from menopausal symptoms. Some women achieve relief of vaginal dryness by using a product such as Replens.™ This is a vaginal moisturizer containing polycarbophil, which can hold up to 60 times its weight in water. The gel clings to the walls of the vagina and water is gradually released into the walls. It can take up to three weeks of use for women to notice an effect. The gel is inserted into the vagina three times a week. This treatment is available over the counter at most drug stores and supermarkets. It should be noted that this is not a lubricant and is not intended to be used to ease vaginal penetration.

For women who are experiencing loss of libido after breast cancer treatment, the solution may lie in counseling for the couple. Loss of libido can be very frustrating and may be experienced as a loss for both partners. Understanding the complexity of sexual desire is a good first step, and a sex therapist or sexuality counselor is the ideal professional to work with the couple so that they can reframe their understanding of the woman's sexual desire and work toward creating something new. Basson's model (discussed in chapter 2) may be a useful framework for gaining this understanding. Basson suggests that women may not feel spontaneous desire, but if they are in a good relationship and are willing to engage in sexual activity, then desire may occur when certain sexual prompts occur. These may be verbal (the partners expressing their love and desire for each other) or physical (sexual touching by the woman's partner at an appropriate time and place). Desire may also occur when the woman realizes that she is becoming aroused in response to the words or touch of her partner. The pleasure she experiences from this further motivates her at a future time to be receptive to sexual touching.

Some women find that attending a support group is the best thing they ever do as part of their recovery. There are many support groups available; some of them are even online, so distance is not an issue. Most hospitals and cancer centers have a list of support groups that may be specific to women of different ages and ethnic groups.

GYNECOLOGICAL CANCER

Gynecological cancers are those affecting the cervix, uterus, ovaries, vulva, and vagina. These cancers are diagnosed in 5,000 to 40,000 women each year, with cancer of the uterus being the most common and cancer of the vulva or vagina being the least common. Because of their location and involvement in sexual functioning, these cancers have the greatest impact on women's sexuality.

Changes in the anatomy of the pelvis from the treatment of these cancers usually result in pain, loss of sensation, and loss of interest in sex. Fatigue is a common side effect of both radiation and chemotherapy. Women also experience changes in their sexual self-concept and body image. Let us now look at the different kinds of gynecological cancer and their effects on sexuality.

Cervical Cancer

Cervical cancer is one of the cancers for which, if it is caught early, there is a high rate of survival. With regular Pap tests, any changes to the cells of the cervix are recognized before they become cancerous. Changes to the cells of the cervix may result in bleeding after sexual intercourse, and this may be the first sign that something is not right. Some women may experience fatigue, unusual vaginal discharge, and pain, and this prompts a visit to the physician where the diagnosis is made. Every year 11,000 women are diagnosed with this cancer and have to undergo surgery and/or radiation.

> Barbara, a vibrant woman of 55, was completely shocked when she was told she had cervical cancer. She had stopped going for Pap tests every year when her periods stopped six years before, but she had had no indication that anything was wrong.

Everything went so fast after the diagnosis; she had surgery within a few weeks and then waited to hear if she needed additional treatment.

Barbara was married to Stan, and before this they'd had an active and satisfying sex life. About six weeks after her surgery, they tried to make love. Barbara couldn't believe how much it hurt. It felt as if she was being torn apart, and she pushed Stan away and then apologized. Stan was terribly upset; he was horrified that he'd hurt her and they both cried in each other's arms.

Surgery for this cancer usually involves the removal of the uterus and cervix and may also include the removal of two or three inches of the upper vagina. This causes the vagina to be shortened, in particular, the upper part of the vagina, which balloons out during the arousal phase of the sexual response cycle. Women may complain that penetration becomes painful after this surgery. This is because cervix itself produces lubrication and so the removal of the cervix results in less lubrication during arousal. This can cause pain during intercourse or vaginal touching and can be distressing to the woman and her partner. In addition to the local changes in the vagina, the removal of the uterus (hysterectomy) is known to cause nerve damage in the pelvis, which further impacts on the sensation of arousal. These changes are long standing and women who have survived cervical cancer may report these changes up to 10 years after treatment.

At her post-op visit with the surgeon, Barbara learned that she had to have radiation as well. She told the doctor that the one time she and Stan had tried to have sex it had hurt a lot and the doctor shrugged and said that perhaps it was just too soon after the surgery. He didn't seem to want to talk more about this, and Barbara left the office with an appointment to see the radiation oncologist at the cancer center.

One week later she saw the radiation oncologist, who told her that she would have internal radiation. A nurse then entered the room and went over the details of the treatment, which would be given about two weeks later. The nurse explained that some women have sexual side effects from the treatment. Barbara's heart sank, but she was heartened when the nurse said that there were some things that could be done to minimize these and that she would discuss them at length when the treatment was over.

Radiation therapy may be given either externally or internally (in which case it is called brachytherapy). Both of these treatments also decrease lubrication and affect the elasticity of the vagina. Brachytherapy involves the insertion of a special applicator into the vagina. The radiation source is contained in the applicator and it remains in the vagina for a period of time.

The end result of radiation to the vaginal vault (the upper part of the vagina, where the cervix is located) is extensive damage to the blood vessels supplying the tissues. The vagina does not produce lubrication; it feels dry and may be painful. In addition, scarring of the walls may occur and the vagina may be shortened due to this. The ovaries may be exposed to some of the radiation and may shut down their production of estrogen, further affecting vaginal lubrication. It is extremely common for women to experience pain during intercourse following radiation therapy. Some women also report a burning sensation in the vagina after intercourse when semen touches the vaginal walls.

Areas close to the vagina will also be exposed to some radiation, and this may cause problems for the bladder and bowel. These will also impact on sexual functioning. If the bladder is irritated from the radiation, the woman will most likely experience the sensation of needing to urinate frequently. Radiation damage to the bowel results in pain, diarrhea, and even rectal bleeding. Women who have had treatment for cervical cancer may fear intercourse because of the pain it causes and may also be fearful that sexual activity may cause a recurrence of the disease. There is no evidence suggesting that this is possible, but it is understandable that women may have this concern.

There are emotional consequences from both the diagnosis and the treatment of cervical cancer. Some women may associate past sexual activity with the development of this cancer and may feel guilty. The diagnosis and treatment of this cancer involves invasive procedures, and some women, particularly those who have experienced past sexual abuse, find these procedures very distressing. Some women do not resume any form of sexual activity following treatment, and this may lead to relationship breakdown.

Cancer of the Vulva or Vagina

Jeannie is 72 years old and has not been to see a doctor for many years; she just didn't see the point after going through menopause, and besides, she was healthy and had no time to be sick. Three months ago she noticed some blood on the toilet tissue after she wiped herself. She thought this was a little strange but ignored it. It happened again the next week, but this time it persisted for a few days. She put it out of her mind and went about her normal business. But a couple of days later she noticed it again. She mentioned it in passing to her eldest daughter Norma, who insisted that she see a doctor. This was not as easy as it sounds, and it took another six weeks before she saw someone at the clinic near her home. The doctor examined her and very quickly told her that she needed to have further tests. Jeannie was quite annoyed by this; she'd waited all this time and still didn't know what was wrong! The clinic made an appointment for her to see a specialist, who did a biopsy and a week later told Jeannie that she had vulvar cancer. Jeannie would need surgery soon, and it was going to be complicated surgery.

Both cancer of the vagina and cancer of the vulva are relatively rare, with just over 5,000 cases in the United States per year. Cancer of the vagina is usually caused by the spread of cancer from either the cervix or the uterus itself. Cancer of the vulva occurs mostly in women over 60 years old. The usual treatment is radical surgery, in which most of the vulva (both sets of labia and the clitoris), the vagina, the uterus, the lower end of the urethra, and lymph nodes are removed. This has far-reaching consequences for the woman involved, in terms of body image and ability to be sexually active. But increasingly, surgeons are performing tissue-sparing surgery, especially where the diagnosis is made early, and this has been shown to have better psychological and physical outcomes.

When the more extensive surgery is done, women afterwards report little interest in sex, avoidance of sexual activity, and significant alteration in body image and feelings of femininity. Scarring of the vulva is extensive, and attempts at vaginal penetration are painful. Because the clitoris is usually also removed, pleasurable sensations are absent. A large amount of fatty tissue is also removed, and this can cause pain over the pubic bone if intercourse is attempted. Removal of lymph nodes in the pelvis may result in swelling of the area, and this is a particular problem with urination, as the entrance to the urethra on the vulva may swell and cause difficulties in passing urine. There can also be swelling of one or both legs in response to the altered drainage of body fluids caused by the removal of lymph nodes.

Despite the extensive nature of the surgery and the resultant impact on body image, many women report that their relationship with their partner or spouse remains a happy and satisfying one. This may in part be due to the older age of women who have this cancer or due to the adaptation that many couples make in the face of a life-threatening cancer.

Ovarian Cancer

Ovarian cancer accounts for over 21,000 new cases of cancer in women each year. This is an aggressive cancer and is usually diagnosed late in the disease process. There is no screening test for this cancer and the symptoms are usually vague: they include bloating, indigestion, vague abdominal or pelvic pain, or urinary frequency.

Rosa had not been feeling well for a while. She told her husband Paolo but he told her that it was just "woman trouble," which was to be expected at her age. Rosa listened carefully to Paolo; he earned the money in her family and he was always right. But still she didn't feel well. She waited till the end of the summer before she went to the clinic. Her English was not very good and she wanted her daughter Rosalita to go with her; Rosalita was training to be a nurse and spoke good English.

At the clinic she was examined by a young doctor, whose face changed as she felt Rosa's stomach. She asked Rosa a number of times to describe what she had been feeling. She sent Rosa for a CT scan that same afternoon. Rosalita came with her, and Rosa could see that her daughter was worried, very worried. After the CT scan, she had some blood drawn and then they waited a long time to see the young doctor again. She looked nervous and she had an older doctor with her. They started to talk, and Rosa saw her daughter start to cry. Rosa didn't understand much of what the doctors were saying, but Rosalita understood and afterward told her mother: "You have cancer, mamma. It's in your ovary. You're gonna need surgery."

The treatment usually involves surgery to remove the ovaries and uterus. If there is any cancer outside of the ovaries, this will also be removed, along with some lymph nodes and part of the omentum, which is tissue that lines the abdominal cavity. The resultant loss of ovarian hormones results in the sudden onset of menopausal symptoms that are usually much more severe than those that would normally be experienced. These symptoms include vaginal dryness, hot flashes, irritability, fatigue, and urinary tract infections. The loss of the androgens produced by the ovaries leads to fatigue and loss of libido.

> Rosa felt bad after the surgery. She really didn't want to have the surgery; in her family they believed that it was not good to cut out things from the body. But Rosalita told her that she had to have it, and Rosalita was almost a nurse and knew what was best. Paolo didn't say much; he was a man of few words. He did get mad at Rosa one night about five weeks after the surgery when she told him she didn't want to have sex. Paolo had always wanted sex three times a week; he'd stayed away after the surgery, but now it was time. And Paolo was used to getting what he wanted from her.

The extensive surgery is often followed by chemotherapy, which may be given directly into the abdominal cavity. The chemotherapy is difficult to cope with due to its toxic effects, and many women are unable to complete all their doses. Due to the chemotherapy, they commonly experience severe fatigue, which may last for an extended period of time after the chemotherapy is over. Other consequences of the treatment include changes in body image, including the loss of all hair on the body. This is a cancer with a high mortality rate, and women are often more concerned about the very real threat of death than they are about changes in their sex life. But younger women with this cancer do have concerns about its effect on their sexual desirability after treatment.

> Rosa had the chemotherapy, which made her feel sicker than she had ever been in her whole life. She stayed at home most of the time; she was ashamed to be seen by the other women in her community. She was bald, and the wig they gave her at the hospital looked like a broom. It was very hot, too. At home she just tied a scarf around her head.
> Paolo had stopped looking at her, anyway. She was worried that he was playing around on her, but who could blame him? She wasn't a woman any more; she couldn't do what wives are supposed to do. So she just stayed at home.

Scars from the surgery serve as a permanent and visible reminder of the cancer. Weight loss or swelling (edema) following surgery and chemotherapy can also affect how the woman sees herself as a sexual being. It is common for women to avoid appearing naked in front of their partner when they experience an alteration in body image, and this can cause distancing between the couple. Ovarian cancer can leave a woman feeling inadequate in her multiple roles as wife, mother, and sexual partner. Some women state that they do not feel like "whole," women, which can cause them distress. Some women may be fearful that a lack of sexual activity may cause problems in their relationship.

Pelvic Exenteration

This is a radical form of surgery that is sometimes offered to women with extensive and life-threatening cervical or vaginal cancer. This kind of surgery may increase survival in advanced cases, but it is disfiguring and has many long-term side effects. In this surgery, all of the pelvic organs are removed as well as the bladder and colon. In the past, women who had this surgery were left with an ostomy for the elimination of urine and feces. But today there are newer surgical techniques: women are left with a urinary diversion and the anus is spared, allowing for more normal passage of feces. Some women will also have a neovagina constructed out of skin and muscle from the thigh. This allows them to continue to be sexually active, although many report a lack of interest in sex and great shame with regard to their bodies. Because tissue is taken from the thigh to create the vagina, touching of the vagina may be felt on the area of the thigh where the tissue came from, and this can be disconcerting. In addition, this tissue does not produce any lubrication in the vagina.

Solutions

It's not uncommon for women diagnosed with any one of the cancers discussed above to remember very little of the information they were given around the time of diagnosis. As with any other cancer, when people hear the words "you have cancer," they retain very little that is said after these words are spoken. An additional challenge to the retention of information is that many women do not have much knowledge of the anatomy of the female sexual organs and the way they work. When this is compounded by a lot of information about treatments and side effects, it's no wonder that many women are confused and unsure about what may happen to them. And a cancer diagnosis of any kind is perceived as a threat to survival, so sexuality and body image are often ignored or seen as unimportant around the time of diagnosis. It is usually when a woman tries to return to normal life after the treatment is over that these issues surface. The woman's partner may have the same concerns and lack of knowledge, and so bringing the partner to all appointments is very important. Some people subscribe to beliefs about sexuality that are not factually correct. It's not uncommon for people to think that sexual activity has caused the cancer or that sexual activity after treatment may cause the cancer to spread.

Details of alterations to sexual functioning after hysterectomy were presented in chapter 5. The same changes can be expected for the woman who has had the surgery for cancer, but this is overlaid with the emotions and fears about having cancer and having to have additional treatment after the surgery. Changes in all aspects of the sexual response cycle are to be expected after radical surgery. It's not unusual for women who have had a hysterectomy to have no interest in sex (lack of libido), to have difficulty becoming aroused, and to experience changes in the frequency and quality of orgasm. There may be improvements over time; however if radiation and/or chemotherapy is part of the treatment plan, women can expect further changes or at the very least, no further improvement.

The solutions to many of these problems require effort on the part of the woman involved, who may not have the energy to address them. For example, fatigue often responds well to exercise, but a woman who is exhausted from chemotherapy and radiation is not likely to want to exercise.

Vaginal Dryness

Loss of ovarian function as a result of surgery, radiation therapy, or chemotherapy causes significant distress and menopausal symptoms. The most effective treatment for this is oral hormone therapy, but if the cancer is estrogen dependent this may not be an option. Local estrogen in the form of creams or pessaries is highly effective in treating vaginal dryness. The systemic absorption is low; however, there is a small risk that some estrogen may go into the general circulation. The woman's oncologist or the woman herself may not want to take that risk.

Vaginal dryness responds well to a vaginal moisturizer such as Replens™ or Liquibeads™. These may help alleviate burning and itching of vaginal and vulval tissues but are not intended for sexual activity. For vaginal penetration a lubricant is needed, and there are a number of lubricants available in drug stores, in sex stores, or on the Internet. The easiest to find are the water- and glycerin-based lubricants. These include KY Jelly and Astroglide and are available in drug stores and in the pharmacy aisles of supermarkets. Some contain dyes or perfumes, and so caution should be taken when reading the labels. Some women complain that these water- and glycerin based lubricants dry out quickly and some find that the glycerin may increase their risk of vaginal yeast infections.

Silicone-based lubricants may be more difficult to find; they are usually available in sex stores and on the Internet but increasingly can be found on the shelves of supermarkets and drugstores. Look for the word *dimethicone* on the list of ingredients. These lubricants stay slick and are not absorbed into the mucous membranes of the vagina. Any leakage needs to be washed off with soap and water. Caution should be used if the person involved is using silicone-based sex toys, as the lubricant will degrade the silicone of the toys. Examples of silicone-based lubricants are Eros, Sliquid Silver, Wet Platinum, and Liquid Silk.

Women should avoid the use of oil-based products (such as Vaseline or hand lotion) and anything that is colored or scented and not designed specifically for sexual activity. If the label states that you should not get the substance in your eyes, that is a warning sign that it should not go in or anywhere near the vagina!

Pain during intercourse (also called dyspareunia) may result from vaginal dryness, tension in the muscles of the vagina and pelvic floor, scar tissue in the genital area, or anxiety about sex and sex being painful. The experience of pain can start a cycle of vaginal muscle spasms (called vaginismus) that can be lifelong. This can affect a woman in other areas of her life and may prevent her from seeking medical attention if a pelvic examination is needed. This is of special importance for a woman who has had gynecological cancer and needs internal exams on an ongoing basis.

Tensing of the muscles of the vagina and pelvic floor is a reflex response to the anticipation of pain during penetration. Women can be taught to relax these muscles in anticipation of sexual touch or a pelvic examination. The services of a pelvic floor physical therapist who specializes in the treatment of pelvic floor disorders can be very helpful. Such therapists can teach women how to relax the muscles and control or prevent spasms.

Vaginal Dilatation

Women who have had radiation therapy to the pelvic area are advised to perform regular vaginal dilatation to keep the vagina open and prevent the development of scar tissue in the vagina. Women should start using dilators as soon as it is comfortable to do so and within four weeks of completion of radiation treatments.

- Women should start with a dilator with a narrow diameter (0.5 to 1 inch).
- They should gradually increase the diameter up to a maximum of 1.5 inches.
- A lubricant should be used to ease insertion; an estrogen cream provides both lubrication and relief of vaginal dryness and may be used unless contraindicated.
- Women should be encouraged to use a dilator at least three times a week.
- They should continue with this regimen for at least three years and possibly forever.
- An alternative to a dilator is regular penetrative intercourse, but for women without a regular partner, this may not be a viable option.

- Women may not be ready for intercourse very quickly after treatment is over, and they may be fearful of pain or damage to tissues, so a dilator may be preferable to intercourse.

Body Image

After treatment for gynecological cancer, many women report that they feel unattractive. The scar from any surgery may be a constant reminder of the cancer, and other changes, such as swelling or weight gain, may add to their discomfort. These women may have the same experience as women with breast cancer and may need professional help in adapting to the changes.

Some women need to hear from their spouse or partner that they are still desirable and attractive, but even this may not help. Professional therapy can be useful in allowing a woman to verbalize her feelings, and this should be done with the partner present. The presence of a professional counselor can help to facilitate the discussion and also to provide some emotional safety for the couple.

After treatment, women may report a sense of physical violation resulting from the invasive procedures and the many examinations that they have endured. They frequently distance themselves mentally and emotionally from their bodies during the procedures in an attempt to cope. But in order to have a satisfactory sexual experience, women need to be connected to their bodies and the sensations that are experienced. This allows women to experience the body as a source of pleasure. Women can be encouraged to relearn that the body can be a source of pleasure through pleasurable touch. A manicure, pedicure, or massage can be a good place to start; these are nonthreatening to most women and do not have to include exposure of the body. An alternative is to spend time in a warm bath with soft music playing, just enjoying the sensation of warm water. Women can use hypoallergenic bath products and lotions and learn from their own touch what feels pleasurable. This should obviously only happen when wound healing is complete. Women can also be encouraged to see a counselor to talk about their feelings of exposure and vulnerability during procedures; this often allows the expression of grief and pain and may be the beginning of healing.

CONCLUSION

The diagnosis and treatment of breast and gynecological cancer have profound effects on sexual functioning as well as body image. Problems are experienced in the acute phases of treatment and extend well into the recovery phase; they may persist for the rest of a woman's life. An understanding partner can help the woman cope with the consequences of treatment, but many women will need counseling to fully overcome the challenges of the disease and its treatments.

SUGGESTED READING

Katz, A. *Breaking the Silence on Cancer and Sexuality: A Handbook for Health Care Providers.* Pittsburgh, PA: Oncology Nursing Society, 2007.
————. *Woman Cancer Sex.* Pittsburgh, PA: Oncology Nursing Society, 2009.
Schover, L. *Sexuality and Fertility after Cancer.* New York: John Wiley & Sons, 1997.

WEB SITES

http://www.cancer.org/docroot/MIT/MIT_7_1x_SexualityforWomenandTheirPartners.asp
This is the Web site of the American Cancer Society and contains a variety of pages on topics related to sexuality in women.
http://www.wcn.org/index.cfm
This Web site has been developed by the Gynecologic Cancer Foundation. It is dedicated to informing women around the world about gynecologic cancer.
http://www.gildasclub.org/
Gilda's Club was established to create supportive networks for women (and men) with cancer and their families. These networks are intended to provide information and support in conjunction with medical care.
http://www.mdanderson.org/topics/sexuality/
This Web site is from M. D. Anderson Cancer Center at the University of Texas. It contains a wealth of important information for men, women, and adolescents, with videos and text.
www.fertilehope.org
Fertile Hope is a national nonprofit organization dedicated to providing reproductive information, support, and hope to cancer patients and survivors whose medical treatments present the risk of infertility.
www.planetcancer.org
This Web site is targeted at young adults with cancer. It contains information for this population that is presented with irony and humor.
http://www.ulmanfund.org/Default.aspx
This is another Web site designed for young adults with cancer.

Chapter Eleven

SEXUALITY AND CANCER IN BOTH MEN AND WOMEN

There are various cancers diagnosed in both men and women that have sexual side effects. These include cancer of the bladder and cancer of the colon. The adolescent with cancer presents some unique perspectives on surviving cancer. These three topics are addressed here.

CANCER OF THE BLADDER

Mona went to her doctor for a routine checkup . She gave a urine sample as usual and the next week was asked to return to the clinic for further tests. After a three-week wait, she had a painful internal test in which a sample of tissue was taken from inside her bladder, and she was told that she had bladder cancer. The cancer was bad and she had to have surgery to remove her whole bladder. It was as if she was in a nightmare but she just couldn't wake up from this one.

Almost 69,000 new cases of bladder cancer will be diagnosed each year. This cancer is treated according to the stage of disease, and many patients will require some type of surgery. The surgery involves removal of the tumor only, if the cancer is caught early. If the cancer is found when it has spread deeper into the wall of the bladder or is more extensive, then removal of part of the bladder or the whole bladder is necessary. When the entire bladder is removed, other parts of the urinary tract may have to be removed as well. In men this means that the prostate gland and the seminal vesicles, as well as the upper part of the urethra, will be removed. As in the patient with prostate cancer, this results in erectile dysfunction and absence of orgasm. In women, removal of the bladder may involve removal of part of the vaginal wall, the uterus, uterine tubes, ovaries, and urethra. Women may then have the same kinds of sexual difficulties as women with gynecological cancer. Radiation therapy may also be necessary, and some people have to have chemotherapy as well.

> Mona woke from the surgery to find herself bandaged from the waist down. She was in a lot of pain and the first few days were just a fog of pain, followed by the relief provided by the pain medication, and then the pain again. But the worst day was when she realized that she now had to pass urine into a bag that was attached to the skin of her stomach. She vaguely remembered the doctor talking about this, but she had tuned most of it out. And now here she was, with a bag that filled with pee and sloshed around. How could you live like this?

If the bladder is removed, the person will pass urine into a bag (urostomy) that is attached to the skin of the abdomen. Newer surgical techniques in men attempt to preserve function by not removing the prostate gland, vas deferens, and seminal vesicles in men and by reconstructing the bladder using a section of bowel. Erectile function and normal ejaculation may be preserved with this kind of surgery. Modified surgery in women involves removal of the bladder only, the internal reproductive organs being spared. There is another option as well: a reservoir for the urine is created in the abdominal cavity, and the person has to catheterize him- or herself regularly.

Sexual Consequences of Bladder Cancer

Removal of the bladder has sexual consequences for both women and men. For women the effects may be global, with reduced clitoral sensation, difficulties achieving orgasm, decreased libido, and painful intercourse. If extensive scarring has developed in the vagina, some women are unable to have intercourse at all. The presence of a urostomy bag interferes with body image, and some people experience difficulties with the bag during sexual activity. Even with tissue-sparing surgery, women continue to have decreased desire, and arousal and orgasm problems. Men who have radical surgery in which the bladder, prostate, and seminal vesicles are removed are permanently unable to have erections and no longer ejaculate. These sexual problems are known to cause a reduction in the quality of life and distress. Even when the newer kind of surgery is done and there is no bag to collect urine, the damage done to internal organs results in problems with erections and ejaculation. This can cause disappointment as men may have expected better outcomes with the newer surgery. Urine leakage may still occur during sexual activity, and this can be distressing to the patient and the partner.

Radiation therapy also has sexual side effects, with men reporting a poorer quality of erections, decreased frequency of morning erections, less intense orgasms, and smaller volume of ejaculate. Women report little or no desire for sex. However, those treated with radiation therapy tend to experience fewer sexual side effects than those treated with surgery.

Body Image Issues

Mona stayed in the hospital for almost a week. She hated having to learn how to clean the bag and put a new one on. Her husband had visited her every day in the hospital, but she swore when she saw what she had to do with the bag that he would never see the bag. Never. It disgusted her, so imagine what he would think!

The sexual issues experienced by the person with bladder cancer who has a urostomy are similar to those experienced by the patient with colon cancer. An ongoing challenge is the change in body image resulting from having to wear a bag to collect urine. Some people feel shock and disgust soon after surgery, and many people report feeling sexually unattractive. Fear of the sexual partner's reaction to the bag is an additional challenge. Common fears concern the appearance of the stoma on the skin of the abdomen and anxiety about causing pain if it is touched during sex. People are also concerned about odor and leakage. These challenges may be worse for women than they are for men.

Solutions

At the time of diagnosis, many people do not consider what effect the treatment may have on sexuality; the threat to survival is seen as most important at this time. But after the treatment is over, most people want life to return to normal, and this is when sexual difficulties become more apparent.

When she was in the hospital, Mona received a visit from a woman about her own age who had had bladder cancer. At the time Mona didn't really pay attention to what the woman said, but a few weeks later, Mona found a pamphlet in her bag with the woman's name and phone number on it. Something made her call this woman, and she came round to Mona's house a few days later.

This woman, Stella, was very open about how she coped with the cancer. Without being asked, she told Mona that she had been very much ashamed of the bag and that she had distanced herself from her husband for almost a year after the surgery. Mona couldn't believe that someone else had gone through the same thing as she was experiencing. Stella was very open and told Mona that hiding from her husband was not a good idea. She then told Mona that she should not be afraid to be with her husband, that things could be okay in "that department" even with the bag.

Urine is sterile and will not harm either the person or the partner. Odor can be prevented with the use of a favorite perfume or body lotion. Using a protective cover on the bed can prevent damage to the sheets and mattress.

Ensuring that the bag or neobladder is empty before sexual activity can also prevent accidents. Different positions for sexual intercourse can also help to minimize leakage. The side-lying position prevents pressure on the neobladder or urostomy bag and the woman-on-top position has the same effect. Incorporating sexual play in the shower or bathtub removes the fear of leakage and is also relaxing.

The treatment of erectile dysfunction following surgery is essentially the same as for men who are experiencing erectile dysfunction after prostatectomy. Oral therapies (phosphodiesterase-5 [PDE5] inhibitors), vacuum devices, intraurethral pellets (MUSE), and intracorporeal injections (Caverject, Trimix) may help men to achieve an erection. There is often a significant psychological component in erectile dysfunction, and referral to a sex therapist may help men to explore other forms of sexual activity if penetrative intercourse is not possible.

> Mona thought about what Stella had said about Mona's husband and about how Stella managed with the bag. Mona's husband Mario had been very patient all through this time and it was his birthday soon. For 30 years, they had always had sex on his birthday. Even when the kids were little or she was pregnant. So that day she prepared. She didn't drink a lot and she found a new nightgown that her daughters had bought for her when she came home from the hospital. She excused herself after they watched the late news, and she went and emptied the bag. She even sprayed around the bag with some perfume that Mario had bought her for Christmas. She tried to get herself in the mood and she joined Mario in the bed they had shared for 30 years. She was very scared, and the first time he touched her she jumped. But she told herself to calm down, and he was so gentle. He could see how tense she was, and he told her that he just wanted to kiss her and that was enough for him. But she felt so bad for him. He assured her that was all he wanted, and that night they fell asleep in each other's arms.

The sexual difficulties experienced by women with bladder cancer are often similar to those experienced by women with gynecological cancer. Pain during intercourse may be caused by vaginal dryness, muscle tension, scar tissue, or anxiety. Hormone therapy in the form of local estrogen cream or pessaries can be used to treat vaginal dryness. A vaginal moisturizer such as Replens™ may help to calm burning and itching vaginal tissues. There are a number of lubricants that are available to help women feel more comfortable with sexual activity. If the vagina is shortened by scar tissue following surgery or radiation, the woman may need to use a dilator regularly.

Some couples may prefer nonpenetrative sexual activity, but many stop being sexually active with each other permanently. This may cause problems in the relationship; however, many couples are quite content with this.

COLON CANCER

Cancer of the colon, rectum, or anus is diagnosed in 150,000 new individuals each year. Cancer of the colon or rectum is one of the most common cancers, particularly among men. The treatment usually involves surgery to remove a portion of the colon or rectum; radiation therapy and chemotherapy may also be given. After surgery, most people will have a permanent colostomy that opens into a bag attached to the abdomen. Surgery may interrupt nerve and blood supply to sexual organs, and sexual problems are frequently encountered. These include erectile difficulties and absent ejaculation in men, and painful intercourse and diminished orgasm in women. Radiation and chemotherapy also have sexual side effects; these are dependent on the amount of radiation given and the kind of chemotherapy given. Radiation given before surgery tends to cause more sexual side effects due to scarring from the radiation, which makes the surgery more difficult to perform; more nerves and blood vessels are damaged in the process. The presence of the ostomy and bag has profound effects on body image as discussed in chapter 5, where colon surgery is described.

Colorectal cancer more commonly occurs in individuals over the age of 60, when age-associated sexual changes may have begun to appear. Men in this age group may already be experiencing erectile difficulties, and women may have noticed postmenopausal changes. Men are more likely to be bothered by sexual changes than women, and younger men are more bothered than older men.

Treatment Side Effects

Gene always knew he would get cancer; most of his family had it and he always believed it was just a matter of time. Two days after his 63rd birthday, he received a call from his doctor's office to say that the tissue they had removed during a colonoscopy the week before was cancerous and he had to have surgery. He was not surprised and went into hospital in good spirits. The surgery was long and he stayed in the hospital for about 10 days because he had an infection. He returned home 30 pounds lighter and as weak as a kitten.

His recovery was slow. Jill, his wife of 35 years, tried her best to cheer him up. She encouraged him to go for a walk every day and she baked him all sorts of goodies, but he was not interested. It was as if a light had gone off inside him and he was a paler, weaker, and sadder version of the Gene she had known and loved. Their life together had changed completely. There was no closeness, no laughter, no touching, no sex.

Following the extensive surgery performed to remove parts of the colon, it is not uncommon for men to experience a lack of desire for sex and also to have problems with achieving erections and with orgasm and ejaculation. These effects are in part due to the anatomical changes as a result of the surgery, in which nerves, blood vessels, and muscles are damaged. Specifically, men may not ejaculate outside the body; instead, the semen passes into the bladder. This is called retrograde ejaculation, and it has a significant impact on fertility, as the sperm do not leave the body and are immobilized in the bladder. Women seem to experience a lack of desire for sex as well as painful intercourse and inability to have an orgasm. For those who engage in anal sex, the removal of the rectum can pose a significant challenge, as a primary component of sexual activity will be missing.

> Over the next six months, Gene slowly regained strength. He refused to see his family physician about what Jill thought was depression. But he was getting out more, and once or twice a month he agreed to see his friends for an evening of poker. He spent a lot of time fussing with the bag that now collected his feces. Jill thought he was quite obsessed with it; he checked it every half hour or so and refused to eat anything before going out anywhere. He was still very thin, and Jill was worried that he was not eating enough. He refused to let her see him naked and would not even discuss how he was managing with the bag.

The most significant challenge for people who have to live with an ostomy after surgery for colon cancer is the presence of the ostomy and the bag needed to collect feces. Like those living with an ostomy because of inflammatory bowel disease (see chapter 5), people with colon cancer have to learn to live with the ostomy and bag and to adapt all aspects of daily living to the presence of the bag. But in addition, they have to live with the knowledge that they have cancer and may have to deal with radiation therapy and chemotherapy and the challenges that accompany these treatments.

There may be strong cultural messages attached to the visibility of feces in the bag, and the cultural issues can have profound effects not only on the person with the ostomy but also on the partner. Coupled with the fears and uncertainty of living with cancer, the ostomy may cause feelings of vulnerability, depression, and mutilation. The area where the colon is brought to the outside (called the stoma) always looks red and moist, and touching it when changing the bag often causes bleeding; this can cause anxiety for many patients and their partners. Some people who have the ostomy and bag report that they continually feel like babies. Their feces are always visible, and they spend a lot of time thinking about and planning the care of the bag. What used to be private becomes very public. They have to carry supplies around with them and control their diet and activity to minimize the risk of an embarrassing accident.

> Jill had tried everything she knew to try to get the old Gene back. Every now and then there was a glimpse of him as he used to be, but the moment passed too quickly and she was once again staring at this new Gene, who seemed like an old man at the age of 63. She missed their old life a lot; they had had so much fun together and laughed and loved like they did when they were in their 40s. Now she was lonely and he was depressed. It had all changed so quickly, and she felt so alone.

The partner of the person with the ostomy may have spent a lot of time providing physical care and support during the acute stages of diagnosis and treatment. This may cause some problems when the partner is expected to make the transition from caretaker back to sexual partner. Because many people with colorectal cancer are older, the cancer combined with sexual problems may signal the end to sexual activity for the couple; this may be a source of grief and frustration. These feelings of loss are commonly experienced by both men and women.

Being prepared for what to expect following treatment for colon cancer is an important step in eventually adapting to the changes in both lifestyle and sexuality. Seeing photographs of an ostomy and the bags and so forth that are needed can be helpful for many people. Talking to a person with an ostomy who is of a similar age and of the same gender may also be useful. However, often there is not much time between diagnosis and surgery for such conversations to occur. In addition, the shock of diagnosis may prevent many from seeking this kind of help. Volunteers from the Ostomy Society often visit people in hospital after their surgery; once again the timing may not be right, and it is important for these visits to continue through the long recovery stage. The challenges of additional chemotherapy and/or radiation may also interfere with adaptation.

While many may think that this kind of teaching would be carried out by professional staff members such as nurses, it appears that discussions about sexuality with nursing staff are hampered by the same biases and barriers that affect all discussion of sexuality. Nurses have the same cultural taboos about discussing sex as the rest of the population, and they tend to talk to young men about sex but not to women and older people.

Solutions

The sexual problems most frequently seen after treatment for colorectal cancer are loss of desire, erectile dysfunction, and retrograde ejaculation in men and painful intercourse and loss of desire in women.

> Jill was convinced that if she could just find a way to persuade Gene to make love again, it would make him feel better. This had always worked in the past; they had enjoyed many hours in bed, making up after an argument or after some sad event. They'd never had to talk much about it, either; it was something that they both enjoyed and they needed few words to get something going. But now there was no touching even, and trying to talk about it was very difficult; in fact it was impossible. Jill had tried a few times and he just got up and left the room.

Lack of interest in sex is one of the most difficult problems to solve. This is an issue that has both physiological and psychological causes. It is also compounded by fear, feeling ill due to treatment, and altered body image, to name a few additional factors. Couples need to be able to talk frankly about their respective sexual wants and needs, and one or both may have to accept a sexual life that is different from before. After extensive treatment and ongoing adaptation to the ostomy, some couples will still find that their sex life never goes back to what it was before; this may be acceptable to some but not to others.

Problems with erections can be dealt with by using one of the oral medications described in detail for men with prostate cancer. If none of these work, then more invasive strategies such as the vacuum pump, the intraurethral pellet or penile injections may be helpful. Permanent penile implants may be the last solution, but the insertion of these may be difficult or impossible due to scarring from the colon surgery.

Retrograde ejaculation is generally a problem only for couples where pregnancy is desired; it is usually not an issue for older couples. For younger men, a referral to a fertility specialist will provide solutions to the challenges of retrograde ejaculation; postcoital extraction of sperm from urine may be performed when pregnancy is planned. Some men notice that the sensation of orgasm is changed if the ejaculate does not flow through the penis.

For women who experience painful intercourse after colorectal surgery, alternative positions for intercourse may be helpful. The cause of the pain may be anatomical, due to scarring from the surgery, but this often leads to further pain in anticipation of penetration. The woman needs to be in a position where she can control the depth of thrusting during intercourse; the woman-on-top and side-lying positions are helpful for this. If intercourse is not possible or desired, sexual satisfaction can still occur for both members of the couple from oral sex and mutual masturbation. Some women find that outercourse, in which the man places his erect penis between her thighs, can be a satisfying solution for both of them. If lubrication is used, many men report that it feels quite natural. The friction of the penis near the vulva may also stimulate the clitoris, and this can be satisfying for the woman too.

Some couples find it very challenging to change their sexual practices after years of doing things one particular way. These couples may prefer to stop all sexual activity, and if both are agreeable, then the lack of sexual activity in their relationship is not a problem. But it is necessary to talk about this and the feelings coming from this kind of change.

Strategies to adapt to the presence of the ostomy and bag have been addressed in detail in chapter 5. These include using a cover for the bag, anchoring the bag with a cummerbund, using a stoma cap to close the ostomy for a short period instead of attaching the bag, using a smaller bag for a short period, emptying the bag just before sexual activity, and wearing attractive clothing (such as silk boxers for men) to cover the bag. The use of deodorizers may mask odor, and bathing or showering just before sexual activity also improves the situation. Avoiding foods that cause gas or odor can also help. Finding positions for sex that don't place any pressure on the bag (side-lying, rear-entry, or unaffected person on top) may also alleviate anxiety that sex will disrupt the bag and cause an accident. But these changes can be challenging for those with arthritis or other mobility problems, and they are also challenging for couples who have always had sex with the man on top and are not willing to be a bit more experimental.

ADOLESCENTS WITH CANCER

When an adolescent is diagnosed with cancer, important developmental tasks may be delayed or may not be undertaken at all, and this can have long-term effects on various aspects of life including sexual health. The major developmental tasks of adolescence include separating from family and achieving independence, finding a vocational goal, achieving a realistic and positive self-image, and achieving a mature level of sexuality. Cancer and its treatment (which is usually aggressive and employs various treatment modalities) threaten the last two tasks; and cancer impacts on self-image, which in turn is related to self-esteem, peer relationships, and sexual maturity.

A diagnosis of cancer in an adolescent forces the young person and his family to face issues of mortality; this is out of sync with the usual order of life. One of the characteristics of adolescence is an attitude of immortality and invulnerability; this directly conflicts with the very real threat of death from the cancer.

Short-Term Side Effects of Treatment

Becky was 12 years old when she was diagnosed with leukemia. In a very short time, her whole world turned upside down. Her family's life changed too; her parents had to spend a lot of time with her, going to and from the clinic and hospital, and her two siblings were left pretty much on their own. They were 14 and 16 at the time, so they managed, but things were rough for a while.

There were times during the long months of treatment when Becky thought she would rather be dead. She had no hair, her face was swollen, and the sores in her mouth were so bad that she could only sip ice water. By the time her chemo was over she looked like a freak, and she couldn't go to school even if she wanted to. Her immunity was really low and she couldn't leave the house. She kept in touch with her friends on the phone and by instant messaging, but it was just not the same. They were out there having fun and she was stuck in the house, a freak with mouth sores and no hair.

Chemotherapy and radiation commonly cause side effects that impact on body image, and this may be even more important to adolescents than to adults; appearance and fitting in with peers are central to adolescents' being and feeling the same as their friends. Weight gain or loss, swelling, scars, skin changes, and loss of hair all challenge their ability to fit in. Adolescents are often quite preoccupied with their appearance, and these changes can contribute to social isolation if they fear being seen as different by their peer group.

Hair loss is described by adolescents as one of the worst parts of having cancer (the others are nausea and pain). For young men, hair is a sign of virility and sex appeal, and for young women it is a sign of femininity and sexual attractiveness. The loss of hair on the head and body can shatter adolescents' view of themselves as well as their self-confidence.

Radiation treatments that target the brain or total body, a common form of treatment for some of the cancers that affect adolescents, alter growth hormone production, so these adolescents stop growing and may remain much shorter than their peers. This has a direct impact on self-image and self-esteem. So too does the amputation of a limb, a common treatment for sarcoma (bone or soft tissue cancer), which occurs more frequently in adolescents than in adults.

Having cancer means missing school, sometimes for extended periods of time. This disrupts the development and maintenance of peer relationships. Chemotherapy often causes the affected person to have reduced immunity to disease, and the teen may have to remain at home or in hospital to avoid infection; this too can interrupt schooling and friendships.

> Becky knew this was hard for the rest of her family. Her brother and sister didn't know how to act around her and pretty much ignored her. Her parents were under strain as well. Her mom had to take a leave from her job to be with Becky, and once she heard her dad crying in the bathroom. There were times when Becky's mom had to do everything for her. That was just so embarrassing, but she couldn't even get to the bathroom by herself when it was really bad. When she thought about it she wanted to cry; she was 12 and not a baby anymore, but her mom had to do all this stuff for her. It was just gross!

Parents often have to provide assistance with everything from bathing to eating and have to attend medical appointments with the teenager. This prolongs dependence on parents and makes it difficult to for the teen to achieve independence. Adolescents with cancer may also find that their confidence in talking to members of the opposite sex is reduced due to their absences from school. Some adolescents may try to gain popularity by being sexually active and in this way gain acceptance or be noticed; this has tremendous potential to do both physical and emotional harm.

Long-Term Side Effects

> Becky got better slowly. Her hair started to grow back and she wasn't so sick any more. She went back to school for the last month of term and then it was summer. She was not going to camp this year, but her mom had promised that she could invite three of her friends to their cottage for the July 4th weekend. The water would be warm by then and they could swim and toast marshmallows and stay up late.
>
> The July 4th long weekend came quickly, and Becky was really excited about having her three friends over. They all piled into her mom's van with their brightly colored bags, towels, and sunglasses. Everything was fine until they got to the cottage and changed into their swimsuits. All the other girls had grown breasts over the

winter and spring but Becky was as flat as a pancake. Her knees were wider than her thighs and her chest was almost hollow. The other girls looked so grown up, and Becky could see that her older brother, Dan, the 16-year-old, was looking at them in a whole different way.

Chemotherapy may damage the brain, ovaries, and testicles of adolescents, resulting in a delay in the development of secondary sex characteristics such as breasts, body hair, or the ability to have erections. This is a visible reminder of the disease but may also impact on the adolescent's ability to attract sexual partners or a life partner long after the treatment is over. Damage to the ovaries and testicles may have a permanent effect on fertility; it appears that before puberty, damage is minimal and the girl will likely experience normal menstruation and be able to become pregnant. But after puberty, the damage may be more severe, and women who have been treated for cancer in adolescence often experience a premature menopause, perhaps even before they are ready to become pregnant.

Radiation therapy to the brain may also affect the production of sex hormones, resulting in absent or delayed secondary sex characteristics. Radiation to the pelvis of young girls may impair growth, making carrying a pregnancy to term impossible as the uterus cannot expand sufficiently. There is often an assumption that treatment during adolescence results in infertility, but this may not be the case. Some adolescents may be able to impregnate a woman or, in the case of young women, may be able to conceive. It is essential that all adolescents are given information about sexual health, contraception, and protection against sexually transmitted infections. It may be difficult for parents to talk about these topics with an adolescent, and parents of teens with cancer are often overprotective or in denial about their child's needs and about normal sexual development when it occurs. Some parents do not want health care providers or teachers to give their adolescent child information about healthy sexuality or contraception, erroneously believing that this will lead to early sexual activity.

The Importance of Information for the Adolescent

There is no evidence that teaching an adolescent about sexual health leads to sexual activity. It is vitally important that the adolescent with cancer should know what sexual changes may occur; this may be a theoretical issue, as many adolescents will not have experienced partnered sexual activity, but they may have masturbated (boys more than girls). Or they may have heard about sex from their peers or the media; this information is often inaccurate. Accurate information is always better than half-truths and myths. Adolescents with cancer want to know about sexuality and fertility and how their treatments may affect them. Adolescents may experience difficulties achieving erections, painful intercourse, and problems with orgasm and ejaculation. These are exactly the same problems that their adult counterparts may experience, but a lack of previous experience puts teenagers at added risk in attempting to cope with them. In addition, these problems will not resolve themselves spontaneously and will persist into adulthood.

CONCLUSION

Cancer has far-reaching effects on both the physical and the emotional/psychological aspects of sexual functioning. Regardless of age, gender, or type of cancer, challenges to usual sexual functioning may be experienced. Cancer is, however, a life-threatening disease, and patients and health care providers alike may adopt the attitude that being alive is all important; quality of life may then suffer.

SUGGESTED READING

Katz, A. *Breaking the Silence on Cancer and Sexuality: A Handbook for Health Care Providers.* Pittsburgh, PA: Oncology Nursing Society, 2007.
———. *Woman Cancer Sex.* Pittsburgh, PA: Oncology Nursing Society, 2009.
Schover, L. *Sexuality and Fertility after Cancer.* New York: John Wiley & Sons, 1997.

WEB SITES

http://www.wcn.org/index.cfm
This website has been developed by the Gynecologic Cancer Foundation. It is dedicated to informing women around the world about gynecologic cancer.
http://www.gildasclub.org/
Gilda's Club was established to create supportive networks for women (and men) with cancer and their families. These networks are intended to provide information and support in conjunction with medical care.
http://www.mdanderson.org/topics/sexuality/
This website is from M. D. Anderson Cancer Center at the University of Texas. It contains a wealth of important information for men, women, and adolescents, with videos and text.
www.fertilehope.org
Fertile Hope is a national nonprofit organization dedicated to providing reproductive information, support, and hope to cancer patients and survivors whose medical treatments present the risk of infertility.
www.planetcancer.org
This Web site is targeted at young adults with cancer. It contains information for this population that is presented with irony and humor.
http://www.ulmanfund.org/Default.aspx
This is another Web site designed for young adults with cancer.

Chapter Twelve

SEXUAL DYSFUNCTION

Sexual dysfunction is the medical term used to describe a condition in which normal sexual functioning is hampered or impaired. The prefix *dys* in front of a word means abnormal, difficult, or impaired. While doctors and nurses use the prefix *dys-*, for many lay people, it implies something that causes concern and perhaps even stigma. However you choose to describe or name something that has gone wrong with your sex life, the important thing is to ignore the name and just get help. This chapter will describe the different ways in which sexual problems are conceptualized, as well as some treatments that may help the individual or couple experiencing the problem.

SEXUAL DYSFUNCTION GOES MAINSTREAM

The year 1998 witnessed a significant event that has changed the way people talk about sexual problems. In that year, the drug company Pfizer released a drug called Viagra (the generic name of the drug is sildenafil). For the first time, there was an oral medication that could help men with erectile dysfunction once again to have erections with relative ease. Prior to this, the only treatments available for men were invasive and expensive; the vacuum pump could be purchased at medical supply stores at a cost of $400 to $500, but it required physical dexterity and its use resulted in a penis that felt cold to the touch. Also foreplay had to be halted to use the device. An alternative was the penile injection, but this scared many men; for most men the penis and a needle do not go together. So many men just accepted that with age their erections were not dependable or ceased to exist. Physicians explained to men that with age went sexual decline and this was just the way things were.

But after the advent of Viagra, even the words used to describe the condition in which a man could not achieve or maintain an erection changed. Previously this condition had been known as impotence, a word that carried with it notions of weakness and lack of potency and hence lack of masculinity. Erectile dysfunction (ED), on the other hand, was a more medical term, suggesting that something physical was the cause rather than a weakness or a threat to masculinity.

The "little blue pill," as Viagra came to be known, revolutionized the treatment of erectile problems. For the first time, physicians felt comfortable talking about ED to their male patients, because they had something they could offer the patients. something that did not involve talk therapy or a lot of money or a referral to a sex therapist. It was easy just to take a pill and, like magic, get an erection. For some men, this was the first time they had had hope for many years. Viagra immediately became a best seller, and sales of the drug internationally reach more than $1 billion a year.

Since 1998, two other similar drugs have been approved for the treatment of ED: Cialis (tadalafil, produced by Eli Lilly Inc.) and Levitra (vardenafil, produced by Bayer). Competition for market share is intense, and each year the amount of direct-to-consumer advertising increases. The patent on Viagra expires between 2011 and 2013; generic (and potentially less expensive) pills will then become available. Attempts are also being made to make the drug available without a doctor's prescription. A trial of this was conducted in 2007 in Manchester, England, where pharmacists at Boots, a large drugstore chain, were allowed to provide men with up to eight pills, after which they had to see their physician. Men traveled from as far away as London to see the pharmacists and get their supply. The Internet has also provided a way for men to purchase these drugs, sometimes without a doctor's prescription. The Internet pharmacy phenomenon has allowed men access to these medications no matter where they live and means that they do not have to have a discussion with their physician about their risk factors or the reasons why they want to take the drugs. A multitude of "natural" remedies for ED also exists on the Internet and in health food stores and mail-order catalogs. Some of these drugs have been found to contain the active ingredient in sildenafil, but this may pose a risk for a man who cannot take sildenafil drug and thinks he is taking something natural and not harmful.

FORMAL DEFINITIONS

There are various ways to look at sexual health and sexual dysfunction. The World Health Organization defines sexual health as "a state of physical, emotional, mental and social well-being in relation to sexuality; it is not merely the absence of disease, dysfunction or infirmity. Sexual health requires a positive and respectful approach to sexuality and sexual relationships, as well as the possibility of having pleasurable and safe sexual experiences, free of coercion, discrimination and violence. For sexual health to be attained and maintained, the sexual rights of all persons must be respected, protected and fulfilled" (WHO 2004).

In contrast, sexual dysfunction refers to a state of impairment in normal sexual functioning. The American Psychiatric Association (APA) defines sexual dysfunction as "an inability to perform or reach an orgasm, painful sexual intercourse, a strong repulsion of sexual activity, or an exaggerated sexual response cycle or sexual interest. A medical cause must be ruled out prior to making any sexual dysfunction diagnosis and the symptoms must be hindering the person's everyday functioning." A key aspect of this is that the impairment must cause distress and interpersonal difficulty for the individual in order for it to be defined as a dysfunction. This is important, because unless it causes distress or difficulties with relationships, it is not considered dysfunctional and a person should not be labeled if it does not bother them.

The American Psychiatric Association divides sexual dysfunction into four categories:

1. Sexual desire disorders
2. Arousal disorders
3. Orgasmic disorders
4. Pain disorders

The *sexual desire disorders* are described as a deficiency or absence of sexual fantasies and desire for sexual activity. The age and life circumstances of the individual must be taken into account, and the absence of desire must result in significant distress for the individual.

> An example of someone who could be labeled as having a desire disorder is a 23-year-old woman who is in a new relationship with someone she trusts and has feelings for, yet she has no interest in sexual activity. She states that she never thinks about sex and has no sexual fantasies at all. This bothers her and she knows it bothers her boyfriend, but she is not sure what to do about it. She thinks that she has always been like this, despite having had three previous sexual relationships. She is able to enjoy sexual activity but thinks that she should want it more.

Low sexual desire is the most frequently reported sexual problem for women. Complaints about low desire increase as women age and with longer relationship duration. The presence of small children in the home, feelings of depression and anxiety, and relationship discord all increase complaints about low desire as well. Most women will at times experience low sexual desire, as it is sensitive to life circumstances. But the proportion of women who report frequent or continued low desire is much lower. And only half of women who experience low desire report that they are distressed by it. Of interest is the fact that women on the birth control pill frequently report low desire, even though this is not present when they are not taking the pill. The birth control pill causes an increase in the levels of sex-hormone-binding globulin in the blood; this binds to testosterone and is thought to lower libido.

A number of treatments have been suggested for low libido, and there is great interest in finding a pharmacological treatment for this, given the large numbers of women who report a lack of interest in sex. Over the past decade, Proctor and Gamble have tested a testosterone patch for women with low libido. In small studies, this has been shown to be helpful for women who have had their ovaries surgically removed. But the Food and Drug Administration of the United States turned down the company's application for the approval of this drug, citing concerns about long-term safety. There is a recognition that once a drug is approved, it will be prescribed to many women, even women who are significantly different from the women who took the drug in the trials that were carried out before approval. So the concern about testosterone may be that women who have ovaries and are premenopausal would take this drug, and the effect on these women is not known. Testosterone has been linked with the development of breast cancer in some studies.

When Viagra was approved, studies of this drug in women were already underway. It was hoped that it would promote genital swelling in women, much as it does in men, and that this would be interpreted in the brains of women as desire. This did not happen, and the studies stopped. Bupropion, an antidepressant discussed in chapter 6, has been shown to help women with low sexual desire, but the effects are moderate and there has not been wide acceptance of this antidepressant as a treatment. Herbal products that claim to increase sexual desire in women have not been tested widely, although their claims suggest that they are helpful.

Cognitive-behavioral therapy is helpful for some women with low sexual desire. This therapy focuses on modifying negative thoughts and attitudes toward sexual activity and controlling distraction during sexual stimulation. Sensate focus exercises have also been shown to be helpful; a graduated approach to sexual touch and eventually to sexual activity increases sexual interest in some women, particularly if it is combined with constructive communication strategies with the partner.

Men experience low sexual desire much less frequently than women, and this is usually associated with increasing age, poor health, and depression. Men may experience low desire if they have a thyroid problem, low levels of testosterone, or high levels of prolactin, a hormone that may indicate the presence of a tumor in the pituitary gland. These are conditions that may need to be treated, and correcting the problem may restore normal levels of sexual interest. Supplemental testosterone for the man with low levels is highly effective but carries the risk of the development of prostate cancer, and so it should be used with caution and with regular monitoring for prostate disease. Men respond quite well to the antidepressant bupropion, which despite being an SSRI type of drug has low sexual side effects and may in fact facilitate sexual performance. Cognitive therapy for a man with low sexual desire includes helping the man to identify erotic stimuli, reducing the response to anxiety-provoking stimuli, and learning to think differently about sexual stimuli. This type of therapy has not been tested widely in men, and there is limited evidence to support this approach; however, it may be helpful for some men.

Arousal disorders comprise erectile dysfunction (previously called impotence) in men and female sexual arousal disorder. For men, erectile dysfunction is defined as the recurring inability to achieve or maintain an erection until the completion of sexual activity. Once again, it must result in significant distress for the individual. In women, arousal disorder involves the inability to achieve or maintain adequate lubrication in response to sexual stimulation, and it must cause the woman distress.

> Dave is 46 years old. He has diabetes and over the past three years has experienced difficulty in achieving an erection when he wants to make love to his wife, Judy. This happens every time, and he is very frustrated with it, even though Judy says it doesn't matter to her. He talks to his family doctor about this and he is given a prescription for Viagra.
>
> In women, arousal disorder may be associated with menopause. Karen is 53 years old, and her periods stopped almost two years ago. Since then, sex has been almost impossible. Her vagina is dry and sore, and this makes even the thought of sex painful. She has discussed this with her gynecologist, who recommended local estrogen cream. But Karen is nervous about trying this, because she does not want to use any hormones. She feels guilty about what all this means for her husband Brian; they have not had sex in more than nine months and she can tell that he is frustrated and hurt by her reluctance to do anything about it.

Women tend to complain about lack of libido and problems achieving orgasm rather than problems with arousal. Women are quite poor in recognizing signs of arousal in their bodies. A landmark study of female arousal showed that women did not recognize the signs of genital arousal when watching or reading erotic material, even though a small probe placed in the vagina showed physiological evidence of increased blood flow and vaginal lubrication. But during and after the menopausal transition, many women complain about a lack of vaginal lubrication, which makes intercourse painful. The treatment of vaginal dryness usually involves the use of estrogen. Systemic estrogen therapy has fallen out of favor in recent years, since the first findings of the Women's Health Initiative were published in 2002. The Women's Health Initiative was a large-scale trial of women taking a combination of oral estrogen and pro-gesterone, or estrogen alone for women who had had a hysterectomy. The early findings showed an increased risk of breast cancer and adverse cardiac events, particularly for women who took both estrogen and progesterone. A great deal of media attention was paid to these findings, and many women became too frightened to consider taking any kind of hormones during and after menopause.

The use of local estrogen applied to the vagina, in the form of creams, pel-lets, or a ring containing estrogen, is the most effective treatment for vaginal dryness. Vaginal moisturizers and lubricants for sexual activity may provide some relief of this painful condition, but only estrogen will replenish the blood supply to the tissues and increase the production of mucus in the tissues. The amount of estrogen that goes into the systemic circulation is tiny and has not been shown to have any adverse effects on cardiac or breast health.

Some women may be more interested in natural or herbal treatments for arousal difficulties. There is little evidence to support their use; however, they are widely advertised and may be appealing to women who do not want to use hormones. The most popular include Arginmax, Zestra, and Avlimil. Argin-max is an oral supplement that contains L-arginine, a precursor for nitric oxide, a substance that is involved in the relaxation of smooth muscle. Relaxation of the smooth muscle is thought to facilitate genital blood flow. There have only been a few studies of this supplement, and two of them showed an increase in sexual function for women. Zestra is an oil that contains many ingredients, some of them irritative in nature. It is not clear if it is the application of the oil and the rubbing of it on genital tissue that increases the blood flow to the genitals or the irritating ingredients that increase blood flow to the area and the sensation of arousal. Avlimil is a tablet that has been widely advertised to improve libido and sexual response. The company that produces it (Berk-ley Premium Neutraceuticals Inc.) has published a study claiming to show improvement in sexual functioning, although the ingredients in the formula used in the study are different from the formula that is sold. The company that manufactures the supplement has been charged with making false and unsubstantiated claims about its product.

Erectile dysfunction (ED) is the most common sexual complaint among men. The incidence of ED increases with age, and up to 30 percent of men between the ages of 40 and 70 are affected by it. ED can be very embarrass-ing for some men; they may hide it from their partners and not talk about it to their health care providers. The most common cause of ED is conditions affecting the cardiovascular system, including peripheral vascular disease, dia-betes, hypertension, high blood cholesterol, and cigarette smoking. The link between these conditions and ED is so strong that the recommendation for physicians is that any man presenting with a complaint of ED should receive a full cardiovascular workup including blood tests and a physical examination to identify cardiovascular disease. If any one (or more) of the above conditions is diagnosed, appropriate treatment may improve erectile functioning. The loss of at least 10 percent of body weight, combined with exercise, has been shown to improve erectile functioning in obese men, and a Mediterranean-style diet for two or more years has also been shown to improve erections. Stopping smoking is also effective.

The most common treatment for ED is the use of oral medications such as Viagra (sildenafil), Cialis (tadalafil), and Levitra (vardenafil). Viagra works within 30 to 60 minutes of ingestion and can be taken after a meal; however, a heavy, fatty meal will reduce the effect of the medication. Cialis is also effective within 30 minutes of ingestion, is not affected by food, and stays in the bloodstream for up to 36 hours. Levitra is effective within 30 minutes but its efficacy is also reduced by a fatty meal. Men will often show a preference for one of the medications rather than another. Cialis is popular because it stays in the bloodstream for an extended period of time and so encourages spontaneity; sex can be attempted at any time during that 36 hours. The failure rates of all of the medications are high, and this is related to factors external to the medication. Many men have unrealistic expectations of the medication and expect to perform sexually as if they were much younger. They may not receive adequate education from their prescribing physician and may not know that they have to wait 30 to 60 minutes before applying direct genital stimulation. They may assume that the medication causes an erection, when in fact it prevents the blood from leaving the penis once the blood has gone there as a result of the physical stimulation. Many men do not communicate with their partner about their intention to use the medication, and they may be met with some resistance if the partner is no longer interested in a relationship that includes sexual intercourse. Some men also give up after a single attempt, if the desired erection is not achieved or is less rigid than anticipated. It may take up to eight attempts with the medication before the maximum effect is seen. Men often get anxious about what kind of erection they may have, and it may be helpful for them to try it a number of times without the partner present, to prevent anxiety from affecting the results. Some men respond better to one of the medications rather than the others and for this reason, they should try each of them on multiple occasions before deciding that they do not work. Men who are taking nitrates in any form for the treatment of chest pain should not take these oral medications. They both cause a drop in blood pressure, and the combination of nitrates with these medications may result in a cardiac emergency if the blood pressure falls too low.

Second-line treatment for ED includes the use of an intraurethral pellet containing alprostadil, penile injection of alprostadil alone or in combination with phentolamine and papaverine, or the vacuum pump. These are of course more invasive and more mechanical but they can be effective. If none of these is effective, a surgical solution, the penile implant, may be possible and is usually very effective. It does, however, require surgery with the attendant risks.

Some men have a large psychological component in their ED, and once they have failed to have an erection, they are more likely to fail the next time. Group psychotherapy has been shown to be effective for some men with ED. Talking about their fears and hearing how other men cope may be helpful.

Orgasmic disorders describe delays in achieving orgasm following normal excitement and sexual activity in both men and women. Men who experience orgasm too rapidly also fall into this category. Like all the other conditions described by the APA, these disorders must be distressing to the person involved. Men who experience premature or rapid ejaculation (defined as ejaculation with minimal sexual stimulation before or shortly after penetration and before the person wishes it) are also considered to have an orgasmic disorder; once again, it must cause distress to the man involved.

Many people have unrealistic expectations of sexual activity, mostly based on what is seen on TV and in movies. In these simulated sex scenes, the man and the woman are beautiful, have great bodies, and fall into bed with remarkable grace. Love making is sensual and often set to music. Both partners are turned on immediately and moan and breathe deeply. Orgasm occurs within a few minutes and is always simultaneous. There is no stopping to put on a condom or go to the bathroom. The correlation with reality is nonexistent. In reality, one of the partners is usually more turned on than the other. Elbows knock and noses are bumped. Simultaneous orgasms are rare. Reality rarely comes close to what is manufactured on TV, in movies, and especially in pornography, where unreal situations are portrayed.

> Jill has never had an orgasm as a result of sexual activity. She is not able to have an orgasm with her partner Rosemary, even though Rosemary is willing to perform oral sex for hours. Jill says that she feels aroused but nothing happens. She cannot have an orgasm even when she tries to masturbate, but she doesn't like to do that; she says it feels as if she is cheating on Rosemary when she does.

There are dozens of books written to help women who cannot achieve orgasms either regularly or at all. It is important to note that only 20 percent of women are able to have an orgasm through vaginal intercourse; most women require direct stimulation of the clitoris, manually, orally or with a vibrator, to have an orgasm. And only 30 percent of women experience orgasm in almost every act of intercourse. Some women do not know what they look like "down there" and may not know where their clitoris is or what it does; men may lack the same information. Many of the strategies proposed to help people achieve orgasm focus on adequate stimulation, the use of vibrators and other aids, communication with the partner, and learning to know the body and the individual's response to sexual stimuli.

> Jim has the opposite problem; he ejaculates much too quickly every time he is with a woman. He has never married but dates a lot. He finds that women are attracted to him, but as soon as he gets them into bed it is all over almost before it begins. He usually never sees the woman again; he is so embarrassed by his problem that he doesn't call or try to see them again. He doesn't know why this happens but it happens with alarming repetition.

Rapid ejaculation is quite common, with 66 percent of men in one study reporting that they ejaculated sooner than they wished. This percentage may be too high to reflect overall reality, and some experts suggest that 35–40 percent of men have this problem, but this still makes it more common than erectile dysfunction. There may be a physiological or psychological cause for rapid ejaculation, which is something that tends to occur frequently after it has happened once. Some men facilitate this rapid ejaculation because of masturbation practices, which often encourage rapid ejaculation because of fear of being caught or because the stimulation with masturbation tends to be forceful to maximize orgasm and ejaculation.

Treatment in the past consisted of behavioral therapy, in which the man learned to delay ejaculation by using special techniques. One, the squeeze technique, required the man to indicate to his partner when he was nearing ejaculation, and the partner then squeezed the base of the penis firmly until the sensation passed. They could then resume thrusting, repeating the squeezing as necessary until the man wanted to ejaculate. The other method, the stop-start method, required the man to recognize the sensation of impending ejaculation and then stop thrusting until the sensation passed. Once again, this required the cooperation of the partner. Since the advent of the selective serotonin reuptake inhibitor (SSRI) drugs used to treat depression and anxiety, it has been known that these drugs delay orgasm. This has proven to be a unexpected benefit to men with rapid ejaculation; taking one pill a day or even a pill a few hours before sexual activity can solve the problem of rapid ejaculation. There appear to be minimal side effects from taking these medications; however, some men have reported a decrease in libido and difficulty with erections.

The final category, *sexual pain disorders,* includes dyspareunia, which occurs in both men and women and refers to recurrent or persistent genital pain associated with sexual intercourse. Another pain disorder in this category is vaginismus; this occurs in women only and refers to a recurrent or persistent involuntary spasm of the muscles of the vagina that prevents vaginal penetration by a finger, a penis, or a speculum.

Barbara is 25 years old and has never had sex. She has also never had a vaginal examination, because she is terrified of doctors and shy about anyone, even a doctor, seeing her naked and seeing her genitals. She is going on a mountain trek and has been advised by the group leader who will guide them that she needs to take birth control pills to control her menstrual periods, because it is not advisable for any of the women on the trek to have their periods while they are on the trip. Barbara reluctantly makes an appointment to see a gynecologist for an examination in order to get the prescription. She is very nervous on the day of the appointment and starts to hyperventilate when she is ushered into the examination room and told to take her clothes off and put on the flimsy paper gown that lies on the examination table. When the gynecologist tells her to lie down on the table and place her feet in the stirrups, starts to cry. He doesn't notice, but in a few moments he is unable to insert the speculum into her vagina. He tells her to relax but she cannot do so, and she starts to sob loudly.

Sexual pain in a woman tends to be a chronic condition that causes a great deal of distress to both the woman and her partner. The pain causes the muscles of the vagina to tighten, and it can be very difficult if not impossible for the woman to tolerate any kind of penetration. The pain and the muscle spasm may prevent the woman from being able to have a pelvic exam.

Suggestions for alleviating this problem include relaxation exercises, guided imagery, and deep breathing. Often, however, these are not effective. Working with a pelvic floor physiotherapist may be beneficial, as these professionals can work with a woman, using graduated exercises and/or biofeedback to help her relax the muscles of the pelvic floor. Using a set of graduated dilators on a regular basis, starting with the very smallest and gradually moving to those that are larger in size, can also be helpful.

AN ALTERNATIVE VIEW OF FEMALE SEXUAL DYSFUNCTION

The American Psychiatric Association's definitions of sexual dysfunction are not universally accepted. These definitions are criticized as being biomedical, with no consideration given to the context of women's lives and also presuming that men and women are similar in their experience of themselves as sexual beings and that their physiology is the same. The APA definitions are based on the Masters and Johnson model discussed in chapter 2 and in that same chapter, an alternative model (Basson's model) of female sexual functioning is presented. This alternative model is suggested as more accurately describing how women experience sexual desire and arousal. Also, APA's definitions do not take into consideration the woman's relationship with her partner and the ways in which that may influence her sexual response.

An alternative view of female sexual dysfunction (called "the new view," see http://www.newviewcampaign.org) was conceived by a group of clinicians and social scientists in 2000. This classification was published as a manifesto and has received support from a variety of professionals since then. The classification supports the reality of life for many women; sexuality is influenced by socio-political-economic forces, by the person a woman is partnered with, by her emotional state, and by medical factors. The manifesto is lengthy, with multiple subcategories within each of the four major categories. This model, although created for women, is also applicable to men, who are influenced and affected by the same factors as women. The classification is presented below, with examples of sexual problems:

I. **Sexual Problems Due to Sociocultural, Political, or Economic Factors**

   A. Ignorance or anxiety due to inadequate sex education, lack of access to health services, or other social constraints, including the following:

      1. Lack of vocabulary to describe subjective or physical experience.
      2. Lack of information about human sexual biology and life-stage changes.
      3. Lack of information about how gender roles and cultural norms influence men's and women's sexual expectations, beliefs, and behaviors.
      4. Inadequate access to information and services regarding contraception and abortion, STD prevention and treatment, sexual trauma, and domestic violence.

   B. Sexual avoidance, distress, or lack of pleasure due to perceived inability to meet cultural norms regarding correct or ideal sexuality, including the following:

      1. Anxiety or shame about one's body, sexual attractiveness, or sexual responses.
      2. Confusion or shame about one's sexual orientation or identity, or about sexual fantasies, desires, and preferences.
      3. Fear of judgment or punishment by cultural, community, or religious institutions.

   C. Inhibitions due to conflict between the sexual norms of one's subculture or culture of origin and those of the dominant culture.

   D. Lack of interest, too fatigued, or lack of time for sex due to family, work, or other obligations.

Betty's situation would fall into this category. Betty is now 50 years old; she has spent most of her life in a small rural community in North Carolina. She was married at the age of 16 to a man from the same small town. He was just 17 years old when they married and within a year she had a baby, followed by another six children, one each year. Betty's mother never told her about contraception or sex; she was also a very young bride and this was just not something that was talked about. Now at age 50, Betty feels different. She doesn't know why but she just doesn't want to have sex anymore. Her husband likes to have sex at least three times a week, and that's what they've done all the years of their marriage. She used to like it well enough, but lately just the thought of it makes her feel ill. Billy, her husband, is getting mad at her. She can't explain why she feels this way; she just does.

Betty may be going through menopause and experiencing a decreased interest in sex because of changing hormones. But she has little understanding of how her body works or the natural changes associated with aging. She was very young when she married Billy, and she came from a home where sex and related matters were not talked about. Her mother probably has the same barriers, because she also married very young. Betty is having a problem in part because she lacks knowledge about the normal changes that can occur with aging. Because of this, and because of the usual pattern of not talking about these things in her family, Betty can't talk to her husband about how she is feeling, and he is getting angry with her response to his sexual advances.

II. Sexual Problems Due to Partner and Relationship

    A. Inhibition, avoidance, or distress arising from the following:

        1. Betrayal, dislike, fear, or resentment of partner, abuse or exploitation by partner, or partner's unequal power status.

        2. Discrepancies in desire for frequency or nature of sexual activity.

        3. Inability to communicate effectively about preferences for initiation, pacing, or shaping of sexual activities.

        4. Disagreements, spoken or assumed, about the terms of the relationship, the degree or meaning of commitment, or the desire for monogamy or nonmonogamy.

    B. Loss of sexual interest and reciprocity as a result of ongoing conflicts over commonplace issues such as money, schedules, or relatives, or resulting from traumatic experiences, such as infertility or the death of a child.

    C. Inhibitions in arousal or spontaneity in response to partner's health status or sexual problems.

Terry and Bryn have been married for 30 years and have three daughters. Over the past couple of years, Bryn had noticed that Terry was less sexually interested in her. She was a bit relieved, as she had never really enjoyed sex all that much. But then she found out that he was having an affair with someone at his workplace. Since then, she cannot bear to touch him. And when he tries to touch her, she feels as if her skin is going to come off. They have been to counseling together and both of them have gone separately, too. Terry says that the affair is over, and that he wants to stay with her and work on their relationship. She knows that his attempts at getting her to have sex are his way of showing her that he loves her and desires her. But she cannot get over her anger about the affair.

Bryn remains angry with her husband because he has had an affair. Even though she has never liked sex, his going outside their relationship to get sex is a betrayal of her and their relationship. He is trying to reach out to her in the only way he knows, by using sex, and this is making it worse for Bryn. She has a physical reaction to his touch, and even though they have tried counseling, both as a couple and separately, she is still very angry.

III. Sexual Problems Due to Psychological Factors

    A. Experienced or perceived lack of choice in sexual behaviors or attitudes, ranging from aversion or ambivalence about sexual pleasure to sexual obsessions or compulsive behaviors.

B. Consequences of past negative sexual, physical, or emotional experiences.

C. Guilt or shame about sexual desires or fantasies.

D. Effects of depression or anxiety.

E. General personality problems with attachment, rejection, cooperation, or entitlement.

F. Sexual inhibition due to possible negative consequences, for example, pain during sex, pregnancy, sexually transmitted disease, loss of reputation, rejection, or abandonment by partner.

G. Deeply held negative beliefs about one's self-worth or desirability

H. Lack of acceptance of age-related life changes.

Amber was eight years old when her mother's boyfriend starting molesting her. She tried to tell her mother, but her mother wouldn't listen. She said that Amber was making it up because she was jealous. Amber eventually ran away from home at the age of 14 and has been living on the streets since then. She is now 16, and for the first time, she has a boyfriend. His name is Matt and he hangs out in the park where Amber sleeps in the summer months. Matt is super cool and really cute too. He wants to fool around with her but she won't let him. She just can't stand the thought of anyone touching her like that. She can tell that Matt is getting frustrated, and she knows that some of the other kids that hang out on the streets call her "the Ice Queen." But they don't know what she went through! She is scared of losing Matt, but she just can't let him touch her.

Amber suffered prolonged sexual abuse as a young girl and is now unwilling to be sexually active with a young man she has met. This is a very common consequence of childhood sexual abuse.

IV. Sexual Problems Due to Physiological or Medical Factors

These involve or lack of physical sensation or response during sexual activity, despite a supportive and safe interpersonal situation, adequate sexual knowledge, and positive sexual attitudes. Such problems may arise from the following:

A. Local or systemic medical conditions affecting neurological, vascular, circulatory, endocrine, musculoskeletal, or other systems of the body.

B. Pregnancy, fertility treatments, sexually transmitted diseases, or other sex or reproductive conditions.

C. Side effects of drugs, medications, or medical treatments.

D. Overuse or dependence on alcohol or other recreational or prescribed drugs or other substances.

Barbara has a drinking problem. Well, that's what her family says. She thinks that her drinking is controllable and she can control it any time. Yes, she has a drink or two most days; her job is really stressful and she finds it hard to relax before bed. So she has a drink or two, maybe a few more when it has been a really stressful day. Her husband Tom says that if she doesn't quit drinking, he is going to leave her. That scares her a bit, but she knows that he is just threatening her. He likes it when she's had a few drinks, because then she gets all frisky and things liven up in the bedroom.

If she's stone cold sober, then he's not getting lucky. So she has a couple of drinks when she comes home. She hasn't told him about the bottle of vodka she keeps in the linen closet, and he doesn't need to know about that.

Barbara is having problems in her life because of her use of alcohol. She is only able to be sexually active with her husband when she has had a few drinks.

CONCLUSION

Changes in sexual functioning are affected by many different physical and emotional factors. Different classifications exist to define and categorize the various kinds of sexual problems that people may experience. A sentinel event in the way people talk about sexual problems was the arrival of Viagra, an oral medication to treat erectile dysfunction in men.

REFERENCE

World Health Organization [WHO]. (2004). Definition of sexual health. World Health Organization [Online]. Accessed December 31, 2008 at http://www.who.int/reproductive-health/gender/sexual_health.html#3.

SUGGESTED READING

Libido

Goodwin, A, J., and M.E. Agronin. *A Woman's Guide to Overcoming Sexual Fear and Pain.* Oakland, CA: New Harbinger Publications, 1998.
Reichman, J. *I'm Not in the Mood: What Every Woman Should Know about Improving Her Libido.* New York: William Morrow and Company, 1998.
Simon, J. A., and V. Houston. *Restore Yourself: A Woman's Guide to Reviving Her Sexual Desire and Passion for Life.* New York: Berkley Publishing Group, 2001.

Female Orgasm

Barbach, L. For *Yourself: The Fulfillment of Female Sexuality.* New York: Anchor Books, 2000.
Heart, M. *When the Earth Moves: Women and Orgasm.* Berkeley, CA: Celestial Arts. 1998.
Heiman, J., and J. Lopicollo. *Becoming Orgasmic* New York: Simon & Schuster, 1988.
Komisaruk, B., C. Bayer-Flores, and B. Whipple. *The Science of Orgasm.* Baltimore: Johns Hopkins University Press, 2006.
Paget, L. *The Big O.* New York: Broadway Books, 2001.

WEB SITES

http://www.femalesexualdysfunctiononline.org
This Web site is intended for clinicians and researchers and contains a wealth of important information. It is updated regularly and has an impressive editorial board of experts who are themselves recognized researchers and clinicians.

http://www.nsrc.sfsu.edu/

This is the official Web site of the National Sexuality Resource Center. This gathers and disseminates the latest accurate information and research on sexual health, education, and rights. It seeks to promote social justice and improve the quality of life of Americans through constructive dialogue on sexual matters. The Web site has links to quality resources and associations concerned with healthy sexuality.

http://www.newviewcampaign.org/

This is the Web site of the group that developed the New View of Women's Sexual Problems. The site has links to other sexuality Web sites as well as updates on meetings.

http://www.aasect.org/

The American Association of Sexuality Educators, Counselors, and Therapists (AASECT) is a not-for-profit, interdisciplinary professional organization that provides certification and ongoing education for those in the field. This Web site contains a list of certified sex therapists, counselors, and educators who may be contacted for help with sexual problems.

http://www.aamft.org/

The American Association for Marriage and Family Therapy (AAMFT) is the professional association for the field of marriage and family therapy. It represents the professional interests of more than 24,000 marriage and family therapists throughout the United States, Canada, and elsewhere.

INDEX

Adolescence: cancer during, 141–44; illness during, 28–29; psychosexual development, 25–29

Adulthood: middle, 31; older, 31–33; young, 29–31

AIDS, 51–54

Alcohol, 78, 157–58. *See also* Substance abuse

American Psychiatric Association (APA), 147, 154

Amphetamines, 78–79. *See also* Substance abuse

Amputation, 85–86, 86–87, 88, 89, 90, 142

Androgen deprivation therapy, 101–2

Antianxiety medications, 74, 75

Antidepressants, 72–74, 75, 76, 153

Antipsychotic medications, 77

Anxiety, 74–75

APA (American Psychiatric Association), 147, 154

Arginmax, 150

Arousal disorders, 149–52. *See also* Erectile dysfunction

Arousal phase of sexual response cycle, 17

Arthritis, 44–47, 68

Autonomic dysreflexia, 94

Avlimil, 150

Basson, Rosemary, 17–18, 122–23

Benign prostatic hypertrophy (BPH), 68–69

Birth control pill, 148

Bladder cancer, 133–36

Bladder problems: cervical cancer, 125; multiple sclerosis, 43; spinal cord injury, 92–93, 94. *See also* Incontinence

Body image issues: adolescents, 26, 28, 141–42; bladder cancer, 135; breast cancer, 116–18, 119, 120–21; combat injuries, 85–86, 88; gynecological cancer, 131; HIV/AIDS, 53; multiple sclerosis, 44; obesity, 57; renal disease, 55; spinal cord injury, 94–95; testicle removal, 112–13

Bowel problems: cervical cancer, 125; multiple sclerosis, 43–44; spinal cord injury, 92–93, 94. *See also* Incontinence

Boys. *See* Men

BPH (benign prostatic hypertrophy), 68–69

Brachytherapy, 100–101

Brain, in sexual functioning, 14
Brain injury, 83–85, 89
Breast cancer, 115–23; body image
    issues, 116–18, 119, 120–21; case
    study, 115, 116, 117, 118, 119;
    sensate focus exercises, 121–22;
    solutions, 120–23; treatment,
    116–20
Breast conserving surgery, 116, 117
Breast reconstruction, 116, 117
Breasts, 9
Bupropion (Wellbutrin), 73, 148, 149
Burns, 86, 87
Buspar, 74
Buspirone (Buspar), 74

CABG (coronary artery bypass graft), 67
Cancer in both men and women, 133–44;
    adolescents with cancer, 141–44;
    bladder cancer, 133–36; colon cancer,
    136–41
Cancer in men, 97–114; penile cancer,
    108–9; prostate cancer, 97–108;
    testicular cancer, 109–13
Cancer in women, 115–32; body image
    issues, 116–18, 119, 120–21, 131;
    breast cancer, 115–23; cancer of the
    vulva or vagina, 125–26; cervical
    cancer, 123–25; gynecological cancer,
    123–31; ovarian cancer, 126–28; pelvic
    exenteration, 128; solutions, 120–23,
    128–31; vaginal dilatation, 130–31;
    vaginal dryness, 122, 129–30
Cardiac disease, 34–40; case study, 34–35,
    35–36, 37; resuming sexual activity,
    36–37, 39–40; sexual functioning
    myths, 36; treatment of sexual
    problems, 38–39
Cardiac surgery, 66–67
Catheters, 43
Cervical cancer, 123–25
Cervix: removal during hysterectomy, 62;
    as sexual organ, 10
Chemotherapy: adolescents with cancer,
    141, 142, 143; breast cancer, 117–19;
    colon cancer, 137; ovarian cancer, 127;
    testicular cancer, 111
Childhood sexual abuse, 157
Chronic kidney disease (CKD), 54–55

Chronic obstructive pulmonary disease
    (COPD), 48–49
Cialis. See Tadalafil (Cialis)
CKD (chronic kidney disease), 54–55
Clitoris, 9–10
Closed head injuries, 84
Cognitive-behavioral therapy, 148
Cognitive therapy, 149
Colon cancer, 136–41; solutions, 139–41;
    treatment side effects, 137–39
Colon surgery, 63–66
Colostomy bag, 64, 66, 137, 138–39,
    140–41
Combat injuries, 82–90; changes in
    access to sexual activity, 88; changes
    in mechanics of sex, 86–88;
    posttraumatic stress disorder, 85, 87,
    88; relationship changes, 88–89;
    solutions, 89–90; traumatic brain
    injury, 83–85, 89
COPD (chronic obstructive pulmonary
    disease), 48–49
Coronary artery bypass graft (CABG), 67
Couples counseling, 107–8
Cowper's glands, 12
Crohn's disease, 63, 64
Cryosurgery, 101

Depression, 41–42, 71–74
Desire, lack of. See Sexual desire disorders
Desire phase of sexual response cycle, 17
Diabetes, 49–51
Dialysis treatment, 54, 55
Disease. See Medical disease; Mental
    illness; Surgical disease; specific diseases
Drugs used to enhance sex, 79–80
Dyspareunia: cervical cancer, 124; colon
    cancer, 140; colon surgery, 65;
    gynecological cancer, 130; sexual
    pain disorders, 153, 154

EBRT (external beam radiation therapy),
    100–101
Economic factors, sexual dysfunction due
    to, 155–56
Ecstasy (drug), 79
ED. See Erectile dysfunction
Ejaculation: rapid, 153; retrograde, 65,
    69, 137, 140

Embryo creation, 30–31
Emotional changes during adolescence, 26
Energy required by sex, 37
Enlarged prostate, 68–69
Erectile dysfunction (ED): benign prostatic hypertrophy, 69; bladder cancer, 136; cardiac disease, 35; causes, 150–51; colon cancer, 140; colon surgery, 65; cryosurgery, 101; diabetes, 50, 51; HIV/AIDS, 52, 53; incidence, 150; mainstream nature of, 145–46; prostate cancer, 98–99, 100, 101, 102–8; radiation therapy, 100, 104; radical prostatectomy, 98–99, 103–4; renal disease, 54, 55; spinal cord injury, 92, 95; traumatic brain injury, 84; treatment, 38–39, 151–52
Erectile rehabilitation, 106
Estrogen: for arousal disorder, 150; breast cancer and, 119–20, 122; gynecological cancer and, 129; as sex hormone, 13; for Sjogren's syndrome, 47–48
Excitement phase of sexual response cycle, 14, 17
Exercise, 121
External beam radiation therapy (EBRT), 100–101

Fatigue, 41
Fecal incontinence, 56
Females. See Women
Fertility: adolescent illness, 28–29, 143; benign prostatic hypertrophy, 69; colon cancer, 137, 140; colon surgery, 65; testicular cancer, 111–12; young adult illness, 30–31

Gastric bypass surgery, 57, 58
Genital area, trauma to, 87–88, 89
Girls. See Women
Glycerin-based lubricants, 129
Group psychotherapy, 152
Gynecological cancer, 123–31; body image issues, 131; cancer of the vulva or vagina, 125–26; cervical cancer, 123–25; ovarian cancer, 126–28; pelvic exenteration, 128; solutions, 128–29; vaginal dilatation and, 130–31; vaginal dryness and, 129–30

HAART (highly active antiretroviral therapy), 52–53
Hair loss, from chemotherapy, 117–18
Head injuries, closed, 84
Health care providers: older adults and, 33; talking about sexuality with, 4–5, 19–20, 139
Heart attack, 36, 37, 39
Highly active antiretroviral therapy (HAART), 52–53
Hip replacement surgery, 68
HIV/AIDS, 51–54
Homosexuality, 27
Hormones, sex, 12–14
Hypertension, 35
Hysterectomy, 60–63

Ileoanal pouch, 63–64, 65
Incontinence, 55–57, 100. See also Bladder problems; Bowel problems
Inflatable penile implants, 106
Information for adolescents, 27–28, 143–44
Intellectual disability, 80–81
Intercourse, painful. See Dyspareunia
Interest phase of sexual response cycle, 17
Intimacy, 8
Intracavernosal injections, 95
Intraurethral pellets (MUSE), 105

Johnson, Virginia, 14–17
Joint replacement surgery, 68

Kidney disease, 54–55
Kidney transplants, 54, 55
Knee replacement surgery, 68

Levitra. See Vardenafil (Levitra)
Libido, low. See Sexual desire disorders
Life span, sexuality across, 25–33; adolescence, 25–29; mid-adulthood, 31; older adulthood, 31–33; young adulthood, 29–31
Lipodystrophy, 52–53
Lubricants, 129–30

Lumpectomy, 116, 117
Lung disease, 48–49

Males. *See* Men
Marijuana, 78. *See also* Substance abuse
Mastectomy, radical, 116
Masters, William, 14–17
Masturbation, 27, 80–81
Media as information source, 27–28
Medical disease, 34–59; arthritis, 44–47;
    cardiac disease, 34–40; diabetes,
    49–51; HIV/AIDS, 51–54;
    incontinence, 55–57; lung disease,
    48–49; multiple sclerosis, 40–44;
    obesity, 57–58; renal disease, 54–55;
    Sjogren's syndrome, 47–48
Medical factors, sexual dysfunction due
    to, 157–58
Medications: antipsychotic, 77; anxiety,
    74, 75; arthritis, 46; cardiac disease,
    38; depression, 72–74; erectile
    dysfunction, 38–39; incontinence, 56;
    neuroleptic, 77; obsessive-compulsive
    disorder, 76; in older adulthood, 32;
    pain, 89; schizophrenia, 77; sexual
    desire disorder, 148; traumatic brain
    injury, 85
Men: antidepressants, 72–73; anxiety,
    75; arthritis, 68; bladder cancer, 133,
    134–35, 136; cardiac surgery, 67; colon
    cancer, 137; colon surgery, 64, 65;
    combat injuries, 86, 87; diabetes, 50;
    fertility issues in young adulthood,
    30; HIV/AIDS, 52, 53; incontinence,
    56, 57; obesity, 57; older adulthood,
    32–33; orgasmic disorders, 153; renal
    disease, 54, 55; secondary sex
    characteristics development, 26; sex
    hormones, 12, 13; sexual desire
    disorders, 148–49; sexual organs,
    10–12; sexual pain disorders, 153;
    sexual response cycle, 14, 15–17;
    spinal cord injury, 91–93, 95;
    substance abuse, 78, 79–80. *See also*
    Cancer in both men and women;
    Cancer in men; Erectile dysfunction
Menopause, 119, 122, 155–56
Mental illness, 71–81; anxiety, 74–75;
    depression, 71–74; intellectual
    disability, 80–81; obsessive-
    compulsive disorder, 75–76;
    schizophrenia, 76–77; substance
    abuse, 77–80
Methamphetamine, 79
Mid-adulthood, 31
MI (myocardial infarction), 36, 37, 39
Moisturizers, vaginal, 122, 129, 136
Mortality issues, 28, 127, 141
Multiple sclerosis (MS), 40–44
Muscle spasticity, 42–43
MUSE (intraurethral pellets), 105
Myocardial infarction (MI), 36, 37, 39

Neobladder, 134, 135–36
Nerve damage, 89
Nerve pain, 42
Neuroleptic medications, 77
Nucleoside reverse transcriptase
    inhibitors (NRTIs), 52

OA (osteoarthritis), 45–46
Obesity, 57–58
Obsessive-compulsive disorder (OCD),
    75–76
Older adulthood, 31–33
Opiates, 78. *See also* Substance abuse
Orgasmic disorders, 73, 99–100, 152–53
Orgasmic phase of sexual response cycle,
    14–16, 17
Orthopedic surgery, 68
Osteoarthritis (OA), 45–46
Ostomy and bag following colon surgery,
    64, 66, 137, 138–39, 140–41
Outercourse, 48, 65, 140
Ovarian cancer, 126–28
Ovaries, removal during hysterectomy, 63

Pain medication, 89
Partners: breast cancer and, 118, 121;
    colon cancer and, 138–39; combat
    injuries and, 88–89; disclosing illness
    to, 29; sexual dysfunction due to, 156;
    talking about sexuality with, 4, 20;
    testicular cancer and, 113
PDE5 (phosphodiesterase-5) inhibitors.
    See Phosphodiesterase-5 inhibitors
Pelvic exenteration, 128
Pelvic floor physiotherapy, 57, 154

Penile cancer, 108–9
Penile implants, 105, 106
Penile injections, 106
Penile rehabilitation, 106
Penis: cancer of, 108–9; changes after
    radical prostatectomy, 99; removal of,
    108–9; as sexual organ, 11
Perimenopause, 31
Personality changes, after traumatic brain
    injury, 84
Phosphodiesterase-5 (PDE5) inhibitors:
    cardiac disease, 38; HIV/AIDS, 53;
    prostate cancer treatment, 102–4;
    spinal cord injury, 95. *See also*
    Sildenafil (Viagra); Tadalafil (Cialis);
    Vardenafil (Levitra)
Physiological factors, sexual dysfunction
    due to, 157–58
Physiological readiness phase of sexual
    response cycle, 17
Plateau phase of sexual response cycle, 14
Political factors, sexual dysfunction due
    to, 155–56
Poppers, 79. *See also* Substance abuse
Posttraumatic stress disorder (PTSD),
    85, 87, 88
Priapism, 77, 106
Progesterone, 13
Prolactin, 12, 13
Prostate, 12
Prostate cancer, 97–108; androgen
    deprivation therapy, 101–2; case study,
    97–98, 99–100, 102, 104–5, 106;
    cryosurgery, 101; diagnosis, 97–98;
    radiation therapy, 100–101, 104;
    radical prostatectomy, 98–100,
    103–4; solutions, 102–8
Prostatectomy, 69, 98–100, 103–4
Prostate-specific antigen (PSA)
    screening, 97
Psychogenic erections, 92
Psychological factors, sexual dysfunction
    due to, 156–57
PTSD (posttraumatic stress disorder),
    85, 87, 88
Pubic mound, 9

Radiation therapy: adolescents with
    cancer, 141–42, 143; bladder cancer,
134–35; breast cancer, 118; cervical
    cancer, 124–25; colon cancer, 137;
    prostate cancer, 100–101, 104;
    testicular cancer, 111
Radical mastectomy, 116
Radical prostatectomy, 98–100, 103–4
RA (rheumatoid arthritis), 45, 46
Rectum, surgical removal of, 63, 64
Reflex erections, 92
Refractory period, 16–17
Relationships. *See* Partners
Renal disease, 54–55
Replens, 122, 129, 136
Resolution phase of sexual response cycle,
    16–17
Retrograde ejaculation, 65, 69, 137, 140
Rheumatoid arthritis (RA), 45, 46
"Roto-rooter procedure," 68–69

SAD (social anxiety disorder), 74
Satisfaction phase of sexual response
    cycle, 17
Schizophrenia, 76–77
Scripts, sexual, 18–19
Scrotum, 11
Secondary sex characteristics, 25–26
Selective serotonin reuptake inhibitors
    (SSRIs), 72–73, 74, 75, 76, 153
Self-esteem, 26, 28
Seminal vesicles, 11–12
Semi-rigid penile implants, 106
Sensate focus exercises, 121–22
Serotonin-2 receptor blockers, 73
Sex, drugs used to enhance, 79–80
Sex hormones, 12–14
Sex therapists, talking about sex with, 20
Sexual abuse, 80, 81, 157
Sexual activity during adolescence, 27
Sexual anatomy, 9–12
Sexual attractions during adolescence, 27
Sexual challenges, dealing with, 4–5
Sexual desire disorders: breast cancer,
    122–23; colon cancer, 139–40;
    depression, 72–73; HIV/AIDS, 52;
    renal disease, 54, 55; sexual
    dysfunction, 147–49
Sexual dysfunction, 145–59; alternative
    view of female sexual dysfunction,
    154–58; arousal disorders, 149–52;

categories, 147–54; defined, 9, 147, 154; mainstream nature of, 145–46; orgasmic disorders, 152–53; partner/relationship factors, 156; physiological/medical factors, 157–58; psychological factors, 156–57; sexual desire disorders, 147–49; sexual pain disorders, 153–54; sociocultural/political/economic factors, 155–56

Sexual functioning, 8–22; brain in, 14; defined, 9; hormonal influences, 12–14; humans as sexual beings, 18–19; sexual anatomy, 9–12; sexual response cycle, 14–18; talking about sex, 4–5, 19–20, 139

Sexual health, 146–47

Sexuality: across life span, 25–33; defined, 8–9; importance of, 3, 4

Sexuality counselors, talking about sex with, 20

Sexually intrusive behaviors, 83–84

Sexual organs, 9–12

Sexual pain disorders, 153–54

Sexual response cycle, 14–18

Sexual scripts, 18–19

Sildenafil (Viagra): arousal disorders, 151; Ecstasy (drug) and, 79; prostate cancer treatment, 103; sexual dysfunction, 145–46; spinal cord injury, 95; for women, 148. See also Phosphodiesterase-5 inhibitors

Silicone-based lubricants, 129–30

Singer Kaplan, Helen, 17

Sjogren's syndrome, 47–48

Social anxiety disorder (SAD), 74

Social changes during adolescence, 26

Sociocultural factors, sexual dysfunction due to, 155–56

Spasticity, 42–43

Spectatoring, 75

Sperm banking, 30, 112

Spinal cord injury, 91–96; body image issues, 94–95; effects on men, 91–93, 95; effects on women, 93–94, 95; solutions, 95

Spouses. See Partners

Squeeze technique, 153

SSRIs. See Selective serotonin reuptake inhibitors

Steroids, 46

Stoma, following colon surgery, 64, 66, 138

Stop-start method, 153

Stress incontinence, 55, 56

Substance abuse, 77–80, 157–58

Support groups, breast cancer, 123

Surgery: bladder cancer, 133–34; cancer of the vulva or vagina, 125–26, 128; cervical cancer, 124; colon cancer, 137; ovarian cancer, 127, 128

Surgical disease, 60–70; benign prostatic hypertrophy, 68–69; cardiac surgery, 66–67; colon surgery, 63–66; hysterectomy, 60–63; orthopedic surgery, 68

Tadalafil (Cialis), 103, 146, 151. See also Phosphodiesterase-5 inhibitors

Talking about sex, 4–5, 19–20, 139

Tamoxifen, 119–20

TBI (traumatic brain injury), 83–85, 89

Testicles: cancer of, 109–13; removal of, 101, 110; as sexual organ, 11

Testicular cancer, 109–13

Testosterone, 13, 148, 149

Transurethral resection of the prostate (TURP), 68–69

Traumatic brain injury (TBI), 83–85, 89

Trauma to genital area, 87–88, 89

Tricyclic antidepressants, 72, 73

TURP (transurethral resection of the prostate), 68–69

Ulcerative colitis, 63–64

Urge incontinence, 55, 56

Urostomy, 134, 135–36

Uterus, removal of, 61–63

Vacuum pump, 95, 105

Vagina: cancer of the, 125–26; as sexual organ, 10

Vaginal dilatation, 130–31, 154

Vaginal dryness: arousal disorder, 150; breast cancer, 122; cardiac disease, 38; diabetes, 50, 51; gynecological cancer, 129–30; HIV/AIDS, 53–54; Sjogren's syndrome, 47–48

Vaginal moisturizers, 122, 129, 136
Vaginismus, 130, 153, 154
Vardenafil (Levitra): arousal disorders,
    151; erectile dysfunction, 146;
    prostate cancer treatment, 103–4;
    spinal cord injury, 95. *See also*
    Phosphodiesterase-5 inhibitors
Vas deferens, 11
Viagra. *See* Sildenafil (Viagra)
Vulva: cancer of the, 125–26; as sexual
    organ, 9–10

Water-based lubricants, 129
Weight gain, from chemotherapy, 119
Wellbutrin, 73, 148, 149
WHO (World Health Organization),
    8–9, 146–47
Women: antidepressants, 73, 74; anxiety,
    75; arousal disorder, 149–50;
    arthritis, 68; bladder cancer, 133–34,
    135, 136; cardiac surgery, 67; colon
    cancer, 137–38; colon surgery, 64,
    65–66; combat injuries, 86–87;

depression, 72; diabetes, 50; fertility
    issues in young adulthood, 30–31;
    HIV/AIDS, 52, 53–54; incontinence,
    55–56, 57; obesity, 57; older
    adulthood, 32–33; orgasmic disorders,
    152–53; renal disease, 54, 55;
    secondary sex characteristics
    development, 25–26; sex hormones,
    12, 13; sexual desire disorders, 147–48;
    sexual dysfunction, alternative view
    of, 154–58; sexual organs, 9–10;
    sexual pain disorders, 153–54; sexual
    response cycle, 14–15, 17–18; spinal
    cord injury, 93–94, 95; substance
    abuse, 79, 80. *See also* Cancer in both
    men and women; Cancer in women
Women's Health Initiative, 149–50
World Health Organization (WHO),
    8–9, 146–47

Young adulthood, 29–31

Zestra, 150

About the Author

ANNE KATZ is the sexuality counselor at CancerCare Manitoba and an adjunct professor at the University of Manitoba. She is an active member of The American Association of Sex Educators, Counselors and Therapists (AASECT) and the Association of Women's Health, Obstetric & Neonatal Nurses (AWHONN). Dr Katz is the editor of *Nursing for Women's Health* and writes a column called "Sexually Speaking" in the *American Journal of Nursing*. She is the author of the award-winning textbook *Breaking the Silence on Cancer and Sexuality* as well as *Woman Cancer Sex*. Katz has given lectures across North America on the topic of sexuality and illness.